ADA ENGLISH

Liam,

le gach dea ghuí

Brendán

(2014)

ADA ENGLISH
Patriot and Psychiatrist

BRENDAN KELLY

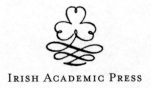

IRISH ACADEMIC PRESS

First published in 2014 by Irish Academic Press
8 Chapel Lane,
Sallins,
Co. Kildare,
Ireland

© 2014 Brendan Kelly

www.iap.ie

British Library Cataloguing in Publication Data
An entry can be found on request

ISBN 978-07165-3269-9 (paper)
ISBN 978-07165-3270-5 (cloth)
ISBN 978-07165-3271-2 (PDF)

Library of Congress Cataloging-in-Publication Data
An entry can be found on request

Printed in Ireland by SPRINT-print Ltd

This book is dedicated to
Regina, Eoin, and Isabel

CONTENTS

ACKNOWLEDGEMENTS

I am very grateful for the assistance and support of Dr Mary Davoren, Dr Eugene Breen, Professor Oonagh Walsh (Glasgow Caledonian University), Dr Ciara Breathnach (University of Limerick), Dr Anne Mac Lellan, Dr Larkin Feeney, Ms Alison Bohan, Ms Joan Patricia Murphy, Mr Peter Finnerty, Mr Colm Croffy, Ms Pat Johnston, Mr Declan Kelly, Councillor Ruth Illingworth, Ms Harriet Wheelock (Heritage Centre, Royal College of Physicians of Ireland), Mr Francis Maunze (Royal College of Psychiatrists), Mr Brian Donnelly (National Archives of Ireland), Mr Brian Crowley (Pearse Museum/OPW), Ms Avice-Claire McGovern (National Library of Ireland), Mr Seamus Helferty (UCD Archives, University College Dublin), *Connacht Tribune, Roscommon Herald,* Military Archives (Cathal Brugha Barracks, Dublin), Kenny's Bookshop and Art Gallery (Galway), Town Hall Theatre (Galway), Dr John Bruzzi, Professor Patricia Casey (University College Dublin), Dr John Sheehan (Mater Misericordiae University Hospital, Dublin) and Dr Aidan Collins (St Vincent's Hospital, Fairview, Dublin).

I am especially grateful to Dr Margaret Ó hÓgartaigh whose publications and support have been especially valuable for this project.

I am very grateful to Professor Diarmaid Ferriter, Professor of Modern Irish History, School of History and Archives, University College Dublin, for writing the Foreword. I am very grateful to Dr Larkin Feeney and Professor Oonagh Walsh for reading and commenting on an earlier version of this manuscript.

I am particularly grateful to Ms Natalie Sherrard for her input into the English family history, in conjunction with Dr Ada English's relatives, and to Ms Úna Fowler for her general encouragement.

I owe particular debts of gratitude to Ms Úna Spain (for her assistance with the images) and to Dr Liam K. Hanniffy, MB BCh BAO FRCPsych (Resident Medical Superintendent-Chief Psychiatrist MHB, Assistant Inspector of Mental Hospitals [Retired]).

I am very grateful to Lisa Hyde, Colin Eustace and the staff at Irish Academic Press.

Quotation from the *Irish Times* are used by kind permission of the *Irish Times*. Quotations from the Minutes of the Proceedings of the Committee of Management of Ballinasloe District Lunatic Asylum and the Minutes of the Meeting of the Commissioner Administering the Affairs of the Ballinasloe

Mental Hospital are taken from the Minute Books in the archives at St Brigid's Hospital, Ballinasloe, County Galway, Ireland. I am deeply grateful to Mr John Dair, Mr Adrian Ahern and Dr Kieran Power for their cooperation and assistance.

Quotations from the Official Report of Dáil Éireann and Official Report of Seanad Éireann are Copyright Houses of Oireachtas.

Quotations from Edward Boyd Barrett's paper. 'Modern Psycho-therapy and our Asylums' (*Studies*, 13, 49, March 1924, pp.9–43) are reproduced by kind permission of the editor of *Studies: An Irish Quarterly Review*.

The passage from *All in the Blood: A Memoir of the Plunkett Family, the 1916 Rising and the War of Independence* by Geraldine Plunkett Dillon (ed. Honor O Brolchain) (Dublin 2006) is reproduced by kind permission of the publishers A. & A. Farmar.

Material from the *Journal of Mental Science* is reproduced by kind permission of the Royal College of Psychiatrists.

Material from *Revolutionary Woman: My Fight for Ireland's Freedom* by K. Clarke (edited by H. Litton) (Dublin 1991) is reproduced by kind permission of the O'Brien Press.

Some of the material in this book was previously published as:

- M. Davoren, E.G. Breen and B.D. Kelly, 'Dr Adeline English: Revolutionising Politics and Psychiatry in Ireland', *Irish Psychiatrist*, 10. 4 (Winter 2009), pp.260–2.
- M. Davoren, E.G. Breen and B.D. Kelly, 'Dr Ada English: Patriot and Psychiatrist in Early Twentieth-Century Ireland', *Irish Journal of Psychological Medicine*, 28, 2 (June 2011), pp.91–6.

I am very grateful to my co-authors and the editors and publishers of both journals for permitting use of this material in this book.

All reasonable efforts have been made to contact the copyright holders for text and images used in this book. If any have been omitted, please contact the publisher and appropriate arrangements will be made.

I owe a long-standing debt of gratitude to my teachers at Scoil Chaitríona, Renmore, Galway; St Joseph's Patrician College, Nun's Island, Galway (especially my history teacher, Mr Ciaran Doyle); and the School of Medicine at NUI Galway.

Finally, and above all else, I greatly appreciate the support of my wife (Regina), children (Eoin and Isabel), parents (Mary and Desmond), sisters (Sinéad and Niamh) and niece (Aoife).

LIST OF PLATES

1. Loreto Convent, Longford Road, Mullingar, Co Westmeath, where English attended for her secondary schooling.
    Source:© National Inventory of Architectural Heritage. Used with permission.

2. The Seal of the Catholic University School of Medicine, where English pursued her medical studies, graduating from the Royal University in 1903.
    Source: Meenan, F.O.C., Cecilia Street: The Catholic University School of Medicine, 1855-1931 (Dublin: Gill and Macmillan, 1987). Used with permission.

3. The Dissecting Room at the Catholic University School of Medicine c.1900, where English attended.
    Source: Meenan, F.O.C., Cecilia Street: The Catholic University School of Medicine, 1855-1931 (Dublin: Gill and Macmillan, 1987). Used with permission.

4. Plaque on the restored building in Cecilia Street which originally housed the Medical School Ada English attended.
    Source: Meenan, F.O.C., Cecilia Street: The Catholic University School of Medicine, 1855-1931 (Dublin: Gill and Macmillan, 1987). Used with permission.

5. English, photographed attending a Gaelic League national convention in Galway in 1913. English (with no hat) is in the second row from the front, beside Máire Ní Chinnéide (with hat) and behind Eoin McNeill (seated in the front row, holding a book). Douglas Hyde is seated to Eoin McNeil's right.
    Source: Courtesy of the Curran family.

6. Staff at Ballinasloe District Asylum with English at the front centre (c.1917).
    Source: Mattie Ganly. Used with permission.

7. Ballinasloe Mental Hospital Camogie Team, 1928. Silver medalists in the 2nd Tailteann Games, Dublin, 1928.

    Back Row: Dennis Coen, Kattie Manning, Annie Egan, Mary Shaughnessy, Delia Kilalea, Thomas Mulrenan, Peg Clarke, Katie Dolan, Mary Norton, Bill Burke.

    Front Row: Bridie Byrnes, Margaret Lyons, Mary Coghlan, Nell Mahon (captain), Dr Ada English, Mary E. Carroll, Winnie Clarke, Annie Finnerty, Nora King.

Original photo by: Central Studios, 13 Nth. Earl St., Dublin.
Source: Ballinasloe Photo Gallery. Courtesy of Dr Damian Mac Con Uladh, Greece.

8. Share Certificate, signed by English. On 22 January 1912, English purchased shares in Patrick Pearse's school, Scoil Éanna Ltd., in an unsuccessful attempt to shore up the finance of the school. Within months, the company was in liquidation and investors only got 6d in the £ in respect of their donation.
   Source: Courtesy of the Pearse Museum/OPW.

9. Cathal Brugha (1874-1922) by John F Kelly (Leinster House, Dublin). Brugha and English found common cause opposing the Anglo-Irish Treaty (1921) during the Civil War (1922-23).
   Source: Image provided courtesy of the Houses of the Oireachtas.

10. Extract from War Office "Castle File No. 4168: Dr English, Ada" WO 35/206/75.
    Source: Courtesy of The National Archives, Kew, Surrey, TW9 4DU, UK.

11. Asylum, Ballinasloe, Co Galway (1900-1920). English worked here for three decades, from 1904 onwards, finally becoming Resident Medical Superintendent in 1941.
    Source: Eason Collection. Courtesy of the National Library of Ireland.

12. Dr Kathleen Lynn (1874-1955), co-founder of St Ultan's Hospital (1919) and Sinn Féin member of the Fourth Dáil (1923-27), who devoted her medical career to the care of infants and children, and the cause of public health.
    Source: Reproduced by kind permission of the Royal College of Physicians of Ireland

13. Dr Dorothy Price (1890-1954) served as a medical officer to a Cork brigade of the Irish Republican Army in the early 1920s, and went on to play a key role in the fight against tuberculosis in Ireland.
    Source: Reproduced by kind permission of the Royal College of Physicians of Ireland.

14. English in Gaelic costume.
    Source: Meenan, F.O.C., Cecilia Street: The Catholic University School of Medicine, 1855-1931 (Dublin: Gill and Macmillan, 1987). Used with permission.

15. Dr Eleanora Fleury (1867-1960) (centre, without a hat c. 1897), worked in the Richmond and Portrane Asylums, Dublin and was arrested in 1923 for treating wounded republicans in Portrane. She spent three months in detention.
    Source: St Brendan's Hospital Museum and Dr Aidan Collins.

FOREWORD

It is fitting, as we reflect on the centenary of many of the events and personalities that were central to Irish political, social and cultural independence movements, that there is a determination to rescue from the historical margins those who have been unjustly neglected. This is particularly true of the women who were heavily involved in those movements, but were also focused on improving the health and welfare of their fellow citizens. Dr Ada English was one such woman, and Brendan Kelly deserves our gratitude for his sympathetic, succinct and clear telling of her story and the impact she made. An account of her life is long overdue.

As an academic, doctor and nationalist, Ada worked and campaigned in a male-dominated environment that was often hostile to female independence. One of the earliest female graduates of the Royal University of Dublin, she was a trailblazer, who immersed herself in the Irish language and Sinn Féin politics, acted as a medical officer to the Irish Volunteers and Cumann na mBan, was elected as a TD and suffered imprisonment. Crucially, she also, in 1904, by accepting a post as assistant medical officer to Ballinasloe District Asylum, began a forty-year association with that institution. Her work in both medicine and politics revealed her strong social conscience, an awareness of the social determinants of health and well-being and her commitment to teaching.

A staunch opponent of the Anglo-Irish Treaty of 1921, she did not voice her opposition to it as the relative of a dead male patriot, declaring 'I have no dead men to throw in my teeth as a reason for holding the opinions I hold.' She believed it was a fatal spiritual surrender and she paid the price, losing her Dáil seat.

But she devoted her life's professional work to Ballinasloe District Asylum, developing occupational therapy to a high degree and promoted sports, entertainment and interaction for patients. These were novel therapies and required insight and determination at a time of overcrowding, staffing difficulties, disputes about administration and management and her lack of promotion; she was not made Resident Medical Superintendent until 1941 at the age of 66. The crucial issue for Ada, however, was a focus on the patients, and she never lost that; at her express wish she was buried alongside her former patients in nearby Creagh cemetery.

As a reformer during a tumultuous period she made her contribution to national life, but her deepest connection was with her patients and her determination to stay in Ballinasloe was testament to this ultimate priority.

Ada did not, unlike some of her contemporaries, leave personal papers reflecting her life and times, making the task of the biographer particularly difficult, and it is to the author's credit that he has managed to locate and distil the public record of her life through research in a variety of different archives. He has also placed her life in the context of other female doctors and political activists to paint a broader picture of a generation of innovative, controversial and committed women who left their mark. They were focused, generous and unafraid to question acceptance of tradition. As Mary Macken, the first Professor of German in UCD recalled, Ada was 'tolerant of everything except incompetence or willingness on our part to put up with it,' and 'she burned to get at her real work of medicine'. This book helps us to understand how that commitment and desire made a significant difference.

Diarmaid Ferriter
Professor of Modern Irish History, UCD
August 2013

INTRODUCTION

————— ℰ ℛ —————

Dr Adeline (Ada) English, 1875–1944

On 29 January 1944, the following obituary appeared in the *Irish Times*:

> Dr Ada English, who died on Thursday last in a Ballinasloe nursing home, was born in Mullingar, and educated in the Loreto Convent there; she graduated from the Royal University. Before her appointment to Ballinasloe Mental Hospital, she served for a period in the Mater, Richmond and Temple Street Hospitals, Dublin. One of the first women doctors in Ireland, she was an intimate friend of Joseph McDonagh, Patrick Pearse, Arthur Griffith and Liam Mellows. She represented the National University in the Second Dáil.
>
> Connected with Ballinasloe and Castlerea Mental Hospitals since 1904, Dr English was RMS there for the past three years. She did a great deal to bring about the changes which transferred the lunatic asylum into the present mental hospital. She developed occupational therapy to a high degree.[1]

As these words suggest, Dr Adeline (Ada) English was a pioneering Irish psychiatrist who was deeply involved in Irish medicine and politics during an especially tumultuous period in Ireland's history.

English was one of the first generation of female medical graduates in Ireland and Great Britain, graduating as a doctor from the Royal University, Dublin in 1903. She went on to spend almost four decades working at Ballinasloe District Asylum in County Galway, Ireland, later renamed St Brigid's Hospital (1960). English worked there during a particularly difficult era in the history of Irish mental health services, characterised by large custodial institutions, which were often over-crowded and poorly therapeutic.[2] During her time in Ballinasloe, English oversaw several significant therapeutic innovations, including the development and expansion of occupational therapy programmes and the early introduction of convulsive treatment for severe mental illness.[3]

In addition to her medical work, English was highly active in Irish political life. She was a senior member of Cumann na mBan (a republican women's paramilitary organisation founded in 1914)[4] and, in 1921, spent several months in Galway jail for possessing nationalist literature. While in jail English was elected as a Teachta Dála (TD; member of Irish parliament) in the Second Dáil. She participated in the Civil War and her strong nationalist outlook was apparent throughout all aspects of her life, including her work at Ballinasloe District Asylum.[5]

The purpose of this book is to outline the life and times of English, and explore her contributions to Irish politics and psychiatry during an exceptionally challenging period of Ireland's political, social and medical history.

Chapter One commences by presenting an account of English's childhood and education, from her birth in Cahersiveen, County Kerry in 1875, through her education at the Loreto Convent in Mullingar, to her graduation from the Royal University as a medical doctor in 1903. Particular attention is paid to her medical education because English was an early female medical graduate in Ireland and her medical education shaped much of her broader outlook in life.

Chapter Two examines English's political activities, with particular focus on her membership of Cumann na mBan, imprisonment in Galway jail, election to the Second Dáil and participation in the Civil War. These activities were not, of course, entirely separate from English's medical activities, and various overlaps between these two spheres are explored.

Chapter Three explores English's medical work, commencing with a discussion of Irish mental health care in the early 1900s, when English arrived at Ballinasloe District Asylum. This was an especially difficult time in Irish psychiatry as the large institutions established in the 1800s continued to expand inexorably, eventually necessitating the introduction of reforming legislation, the Mental Treatment Act 1945, shortly after English's death.[6] Prior to this, English had spent almost four decades working at the asylum in Ballinasloe, where she introduced novel therapies, advocated for more humane conditions for patients, and navigated the complicated politics of asylum life.

Chapter Four discusses English's life and work in the context of four other women doctors who, like English, combined political activism with progressive medical practice in early twentieth-century Ireland: Dr Kathleen, Lynn, Dr Dorothy Price, Dr Brigid Lyons Thornton and Dr Eleonora Fleury. Dr Kathleen Lynn was, like English, a pioneering medical doctor and, in 1919, co-founded St Ultan's Hospital for Infants in Dublin, with Madeleine ffrench-Mullen.[7] Lynn was also a TD in the Fourth Dáil and an active member of Sinn Féin, an Irish republican political party to which English also belonged.

Similarly, Dr Dorothy Price served as medical officer to a Cork brigade of the Irish Republican Army (a republican military organisation) and later played a key role in the eradication of tuberculosis in Ireland.[8] Dr Brigid Lyons Thornton had similar involvements, working with Irish revolutionary leader Michael Collins during the War of Independence and later working in public health and at the Rotunda Hospital in Dublin.[9]

Finally, Dr Eleonora Fleury was the first female medical graduate of the Royal University of Ireland in 1890[10] and, like English, went onto work in Irish asylums, especially the Richmond Asylum (later St Brendan's Hospital) in Dublin.[11] Fleury became the first female member of the Medico-Psychological Association in 1894, at the initiative of Dr Conolly Norman of the Richmond Asylum.[12] Like English, Fleury was deeply involved in the Irish nationalist struggle, often treating injured republicans at her home and hiding fugitives in the large, crowded asylums in which she worked.[13]

English belongs firmly within this group of politically active, socially-minded and occasionally radical doctors, combining strong political views with progressive medical practice, underpinned by a clear focus on improving health-care for the poor, the disadvantaged and, in the case of English, the forgotten patients of Ireland's vast asylum system. Against this background, Chapter Five concludes by exploring English's legacies to both Irish medicine and politics.[14]

Unlike Lynn, English did not leave behind a lengthy diary detailing the thoughts and motivations that underpinned her medical, political and personal activities. Unlike Price, she did not leave behind a trove of letters about her life and times. Neither did English marry and nor did she have children. There are few direct personal accounts of English as an individual. As a result, it is English's medical and political works that dominate this book, as they did her life.

A Note on Terminology

Throughout this book, original language and terminology from the 1700s, 1800s and 1900s have been maintained. This represents an attempt to optimise fidelity to historical sources and does not represent an endorsement of the broader use of such terminology in contemporary settings.

Notes

1. *Irish Times*, 29 January 1944.
2. E. Boyd Barrett, 'Modern psycho-therapy and our asylums', *Studies*, 13, 49 (March 1924), pp.9–43; M. Finnane, *Insanity and the Insane in Post-Famine Ireland* (London: Croom Helm, 1981); B.D. Kelly, 'One hundred years ago: the Richmond Asylum, Dublin in 1907', *Irish Journal of Psychological Medicine*, 24, 3 (September 2007), pp.108–114.
3. M. Davoren, E.G. Breen and B.D. Kelly, 'Dr Ada English: patriot and psychiatrist in early twentieth-century Ireland', *Irish Journal of Psychological Medicine*, 28, 2 (June 2011), pp.91–6.
4. C. McCarthy, *Cumann na mBan and the Irish Revolution* (Dublin: The Collins Press, 2007), pp.173–4.
5. M. Davoren, E.G. Breen and B.D. Kelly, 'Dr Adeline English: Revolutionising Politics and Psychiatry in Ireland', *Irish Psychiatrist*, 10, 4 (Winter 2009), pp.260–2.
6. B.D. Kelly, 'The Mental Treatment Act 1945 in Ireland: an historical enquiry', *History of Psychiatry*, 19, 1 (March 2008), pp.47–67.
7. M. Ó hÓgartaigh, *Kathleen Lynn: Irishwoman, Patriot, Doctor* (Dublin: Irish Academic Press, 2006).
8. M. Ó hÓgartaigh, 'Dorothy Stopford-Price and the elimination of childhood tuberculosis', in J. Augusteijn (ed.), *Ireland in the 1930s: New Perspectives* (Dublin: Four Courts Press, 1999), pp.67–82; A. Mac Lellan, 'Dr Dorothy Price and the eradication of TB in Ireland', *Irish Medical News*, 19 May 2008. Mac Lellan, A., *Dorothy Stopford Price: Rebel Doctor* (Sallins, Co. Kildare: Irish Academic Press, 2014).
9. J. Cowell, *A Noontide Blazing: Brigid Lyons Thornton – Rebel, Soldier, Doctor* (Dublin: Currach Press, 2005).
10. A. Collins, 'Eleonora Fleury captured', *British Journal of Psychiatry*, 203, 1 (2013), p.5; M Ó hÓgartaigh, '"Is there any need of you?" Women in medicine in Ireland and Australia', *Australian Journal of Irish Studies*, 4 (2004), pp.162–71.
11. M. Ó hÓgartaigh, *Quiet Revolutionaries: Irish Women in Education, Medicine and Sport, 1861–1964* (Dublin: The History Press Ireland, 2011), p.147.
12. J. Reynolds, *Grangegorman: Psychiatric Care in Dublin since 1815* (Dublin: Institute of Public Administration in association with Eastern Health Board, 1992).
13. Witness Statement (Number 568) of Eilis, Bean Uí Chonaill (Dublin: Bureau of Military History, 1913–21, File Number S.1846), pp.53–4. B. Kelly 'Irish women in medicine', *Irish Medical News*, 7 May 2013.
14. B. Kelly and M. Davoren, 'Dr Ada English', in M. Mulvihill (ed.), *Lab Coats and Lace: The Lives and Legacies of Inspiring Irish Women Scientists and Pioneers* (Dublin: Women in Technology and Science, 2009), p.97; B. Kelly, 'Female pioneers', *Irish Medical News*, 27 April 2009; B. Kelly, 'The History of Medicine', *Irish Medical News*, 8 August 2010.

CHAPTER ONE

———— ✄ ✄ ————

Background: Childhood and Education, 1875–1903

Adeline English was born on 10 January 1875 in Cahersiveen, County Kerry.[1] Her father, Patrick, was an apothecary and son of Richard English, a tanner. English's mother, Honora (Nora) Mulvihill, was the daughter of Jerry Mulvihill, a shop-keeper.[2] The couple had been married in Listowel on 18 February 1873, when Patrick was aged twenty-one years and Nora was twenty-three. They resided in Cahersiveen and their first child, Lilian (Lillie) Gertrude, was born in Kerry on 12 November 1873. English was born fourteen months later.

When English was a young child the family moved to Mullingar, County Westmeath, where her father worked as a pharmacist. English's twin brothers, Jeremiah Pierce and Richard Plunkett, were born in Mullingar on 19 May 1876. Jeremiah Pierce died as an infant and the next boy, born in 1877, was also named Jeremiah Pierce. Another brother, Patrick Francis, was born in Mullingar on 4 June 1879.

English grew up in Mullingar where her father had a pharmacy, English's Medical Hall, located at 27 Earl Street, in the centre of Mullingar town.[3] English's father was a member of Mullingar Town Commissioners and held strong nationalist views, which undoubtedly influenced English's own political outlook.

English's grandfather, Richard, was master of the nearby Oldcastle Workhouse, County Meath and the destitution that English witnessed others suffering while she was a young child also undoubtedly affected her deeply.[4] Consistent with this, English's future work in both medicine and politics demonstrated a strong social conscience and an especially deep awareness of the social determinants of health and wellbeing.

English was fortunate to grow up during a period when access to education improved significantly for girls in Ireland. The 1878 Intermediate Education

5

Act was passed when English was three years of age and gave girls access to all examinations of the Intermediate Board. While second-level education remained relatively rare throughout Ireland as a whole, and was generally limited to the middle-classes, many girls nonetheless experienced enhanced educational opportunities during this period: in 1879, 736 girls presented for the Intermediate examination and, by 1906, this increased to 3,656.[5]

These changes opened up dramatic new possibilities for further education for middle-class girls like English. During the decade between 1871 and 1881 (when English was six years of age), the number of girls in Ireland studying mathematics increased from 510 to 1,082; the number studying Latin from 292 to 770; and the number studying Greek from thirty-five to 122.[6] These subjects were especially important for entry to university.[7]

English, the daughter of a pharmacist, was an enthusiastic student and in a good position to benefit from these changes. For her secondary schooling she attended the Loreto Convent in Mullingar.[8] The Sisters of Loreto, who belong to the Institute of the Blessed Virgin Mary, are a religious congregation of women founded in 1609 by the Venerable Mary Ward, an English Catholic religious sister. Ward's vision was that the order would be both inspired by the gospel and engaged with the world outside the cloisters. An Irish branch of the Sisters of Loreto was founded by Mother Frances Mary Teresa Ball who oversaw the establishment of several schools, the first of which was at Rathfarnham Abbey in Dublin. Over the following decades, this network of schools and convents extended throughout Ireland and beyond, to India, Mauritius and Canada.

Loreto Convent in Mullingar was established by the Most Reverend Dr Nulty who obtained the site from Lord Greville, a prominent Mullingar land-owner. On 25 March 1881 three nuns came from the Loreto Convent in nearby Navan to take charge of the new school. It began as a day school and the young English was among its earliest students.

In their educational and missionary work, the Sisters of Loreto placed strong emphases on contemplating scripture, identifying with the situation of others, and working collaboratively towards a more just world. This was an ethos which was to remain strongly apparent in the life and work of English as she completed her medical education in Dublin and went on to a life that combined political engagement with providing medical care to the often forgotten patients within the Irish asylum system.

Medical Education

English studied medicine at the Catholic University School of Medicine on Cecilia Street in Dublin, and graduated as a medical doctor (MB BCh BAO) from the Royal University in 1903. At this time, the admission of women to medical school was a relatively recent development and, as a result, English was indeed, as the *Irish Press* and *East Galway Democrat* claimed, 'one of the first women doctors in Ireland'.[9]

The early history of universities in Ireland was not very encouraging for Roman Catholics, such as English. The University of Dublin was the first university established in Ireland, in 1591, and had one constituent college, Trinity College, Dublin. Only a small number of Catholics were admitted initially and in 1637 all Catholics were excluded. In 1849, Queen's Colleges were opened in Galway, Cork and Belfast, but these institutions were unacceptable to Ireland's Catholic majority in Ireland and condemned by the Catholic hierarchy as 'Godless'.[10]

The early histories of universities in Ireland were not very encouraging for women, either. University education for women in Ireland commenced with the establishment of the Royal University of Ireland in 1879, but it was not until 1895 that facilities in all of the Queen's Colleges in Galway, Cork and Belfast were available to women.[11] The University of Dublin (Trinity College) did not admit women until 1904 and even then there were limitations: up until 1930, women under the age of eighteen years were still barred from the study of anatomy and physiology at Trinity.[12]

The Catholic University School of Medicine, at which English studied, was part of the Catholic University founded in 1851 in St Stephen's Green in Dublin's city centre. The first rector was Cardinal John Newman, an Oxford academic and priest of the Church of England who took a keen interest in education and, especially, the establishment of the Catholic University in Dublin.

When it opened in 1854, the Catholic University had fifteen students and faculties included theology, law, medicine, philosophy, letters and mathematics, and natural science.[13] Newman was keen to develop the school of medicine further and in 1854 Andrew Ellis, a prominent Dublin surgeon, purchased a suitable building on Cecilia Street at a cost of £1,450. Over the following years, Newman steadily built up a strong medical faculty, with Ellis as professor of surgery (1855–67) and Robert S.D. Lyons as professor of medicine and pathology (1856–86).

Lectures provided at the Catholic University School of Medicine were formally recognised by the Royal College of Surgeons in Ireland, a long-established medical college, which was founded in 1784 and had the authority to recognise medical courses from other colleges. As a result of this recognition, the Catholic University School of Medicine thrived and student numbers grew steadily, from thirty-six in 1855 to 108 in 1863.[14] The same trend was not apparent throughout other faculties of the Catholic University, as student numbers fell owing to the fact that other courses, unlike the medical courses, were not recognised by appropriate licensing bodies.

The Catholic University was clearly in need of reform. In 1879, the Royal University was established and in 1882 the resources of various Catholic colleges were pooled in order to provide courses for the Royal University in direct competition with the Queens Colleges and the University of Dublin. The Catholic University Medical School was one of the participating Catholic colleges and, as a result, the 1880s saw significant development and expansion at Cecilia Street.

Up until this point, all medical students were male. Prevailing attitudes were plainly stated by Dr Walter Rivington who in 1879 won the Carmichael Prize of £200 for an essay titled *The Medical Profession*. On the subject of potential women doctors, Rivington wrote:

> The profane attempt of ambitious women to enter the sacred precincts of the medical profession has aroused the warmest feelings of antagonism within the charmed circle of regular male practitioners... The professional mind appears to be unable to contemplate with calmness the near prospect of actually existing female doctors... Many of the most estimable members of our profession perceive in the medical education and destination of women a horrible and vicious attempt of women deliberately to unsex themselves – in the acquisition of an anatomical and physiological knowledge, the gratification of a prurient and morbid curiosity and thirst after forbidden information – and in the performance of routine medical and surgical duties the assumption of offices which nature intended entirely for the sterner sex... A few years will demonstrate how little vitality is possessed by the movement for the medical education of women... Woman's disabilities are too many to allow more than a few to adopt the medical profession as a livelihood.[15]

Nevertheless, the Medical Qualifications Act in 1876 removed the legal restriction on women entering the profession of medicine and, as a result, five women were admitted to the Licentiate of the King and Queens College of Physicians in 1877.[16] In 1885, the Medical School of the Royal College of Surgeons in Ireland became the first medical school in Great Britain and Ireland to admit women to its lectures. The first woman student was Agnes Shannon in 1885 and the first woman fellow was Emily Winifred Dickson in 1893.

Some years later, at the Catholic University School of Medicine, Frances Sinclair became the first woman to graduate from the School as a medical doctor, achieving an 'upper pass' in 1898. The following year, Kathleen Lynn also graduated as a doctor, winning the Hudson Prize and a silver medal for her examination results.[17] Like English, Lynn went on to combine pioneering medical work with political activism, co-founding St Ultan's Hospital for Infants in Dublin in 1919 and serving as a TD in the Fourth Dáil (see Chapter Four).

Despite some lingering difficulties, the arrival of women at the Catholic University School of Medicine was generally welcomed. Ambrose Birmingham, professor of anatomy (1887–1905), was asked about women medical students by the Royal Commission on University Education and reported that they were among the best students in the school, were hard-working and earnest, and brought nothing but good to the college.[18] By 1901 there were fifteen female medical students at Cecilia Street. One of these was English, who graduated in 1903.

Professor Mary M. Macken, in her memoir of Cecilia Street, provides a vivid description of English as a medical student:

> I remember her crisp, blond hair, remarkable blue eyes and fascinating lisp. She struck me then as being singularly adult. She was, in fact, some years my senior and tolerant of everything except incompetence or willingness on our part to put up with it. For she burned to get at her real work of medicine; it was for her as much a vocation as a profession.[19]

Although her medical studies took place in Dublin, English was present in Mullingar when the 1901 census was performed. The census enumerator recorded that on census night (31 March) English was present at house number thirteen, Earls South Side in Mullingar.[20] She was returned as 'Catholic', 'not married' and 'a medical student at RUI' (Royal University of Ireland). The only other family member resident on that day was English's mother, Nora, aged fifty-three years.

There were three other individuals present in the house too: Mary Martyn, a 'domestic servant' aged twenty-four years; Mr William James Burke, a 'pharmaceutical chemist' and 'manager of business', originally from Youghal, County Cork; and Mr Francis Fisher, a 'Protestant' and 'bank officer', aged fifty-two. The house is recorded as having between ten and twelve rooms and being located on the holding of Lord Greville, the member of parliament for Westmeath (1865–74) who had donated the land for the Loreto Convent where English attended school.

Following the census, English completed her medical training in Dublin and graduated as a doctor in 1903.[21] She was congratulated on her success in *St Stephen's*, the college magazine of the Catholic University.[22] Ironically, only the previous year, *St Stephen's* had published an 'Ode to Lady Medicals' written by 'Mac Aodh', questioning women's place in medicine:

> Though all the world's a stage and we are acting,
> Yet still I think your part is not dissecting.
> To me the art of making apple tarts
> Would suit you better than these 'horrid parts.'
> ...And as for learning chemistry and that,
> 'Twould be a nicer thing to trim a hat.
> I know your aims in medicine are true,
> But tell me is there any *need* of you?[23]

By 1904, however, *St Stephen's* conceded that female medical students were now 'well known' and caused 'little or no extraordinary attention in moving through Dublin social circles'.[24] Indeed, 1904 was an important year for women in Irish medicine because, for the first time, a woman from the Catholic University School of Medicine on Cecilia Street achieved first place in the final medical examination of the Royal University. Her name was Isabella G.A. Ovenden and she later made an important contribution to child health in Ireland.[25]

St Stephen's also reported significant female activism at the Catholic University around this time. In 1904, for example, it reported that one female student threw a hefty volume of Byron at the British flag above a lecturer, shouting 'Vivient les femmes!'[26] The early decades of the twentieth century would duly demonstrate that university education for women in Ireland had not only provided them with enhanced educational and work opportunities, but would also propel them deep into Irish political life and various forms of social activism.[27]

English was a good example of this. Following her medical education, English went on to become deeply engaged in revolutionary politics (Chapter Two) and devote most of her working life to the mentally ill in Ballinasloe District Asylum in County Galway (Chapter Three). Following her registration as a doctor and prior to her appointment to Ballinasloe, however, English gained valuable clinical experience at a number of Dublin hospitals: she was a clinical clerk at the Mater Misericordiae Hospital, house surgeon at the Children's Hospital, Temple Street, and clinical assistant at the vast Richmond Asylum.[28]

The breadth of English's clinical experience and commitment to education was reflected in her lifelong commitment to teaching: in 1914 she became the first statutory lecturer in 'mental diseases' at University College Galway (later renamed National University of Ireland, Galway in 1997).[29] She gave lectures in Galway and provided clinical instruction at the asylum in Ballinasloe.[30] Interestingly, English's nationalist leanings and political activities were not unique among the university's academic staff: Tommie Walsh, professor of pathology, was interned under the Defence of the Realm Act, and several medical graduates were similarly incarcerated during this period.[31] At various points, Surgeon Michael O'Malley and Dr W.A.F. Sandys treated members of the Irish Volunteers (to which English belonged) and assisted in Clifden, County Galway when the Black and Tans (British paramilitary police forces assisting the Royal Irish Constabulary) set the town on fire on 17 March 1921.

The appointment of women doctors to academic positions such as that held by English in Galway was an important step forward: the medical school at Cecilia Street that English attended, for example, closed its doors in 1931 without ever appointing a woman to its academic staff.[32] The premises at Cecilia Street were succeeded by the medical school of University College Dublin, initially located at Earlsfort Terrace and now relocated to Belfield.

Against this backdrop of medical and academic engagement, it is not surprising that English was an active member of various professional organisations throughout her career. She was, for example, a member of the Medico-Psychological Association (MPA) of Great Britain and Ireland from 1911 to 1921.[33] She was proposed for membership in 1910 by Dr John Mills of Ballinasloe, Dr W.R. Dawson and Dr John O'Conor Donelan,[34] who would later become resident medical superintendent of the Richmond Asylum, Dublin (1908–37).[35] English was to become an active participant in the Irish Division of the MPA.[36]

The MPA was a continuation of the Association of Medical Officers of Asylums and Hospitals for the Insane which was founded in 1841 by Dr Samuel Hitch, resident superintendent of the Gloucestershire General Lunatic Asylum.[37] The purpose of the organisation was to facilitate communication between doctors working in asylums with a view to improving quality of care provided to the mentally ill. In 1864 the organisation's name was changed to the Medico-Psychological Association and in 1894 it admitted its first woman member, Dr Eleonora Fleury of the Richmond Lunatic Asylum in Dublin.[38]

Interestingly, Fleury was working at the Richmond Asylum when English spent time there as a clinical assistant, shortly after graduating.[39] The lives and careers of Fleury and English were to bear further similarities to each other in future years, as both doctors combined medical work in asylums with nationalist political activism, and both were imprisoned for their political activities at various points (see Chapter Four).

By 1901, as English was completing her medical studies, the MPA had 616 members and was engaged with a range of issues including conditions of service, problems with asylum as institutions, and the introduction and evaluation of novel treatments for mental illness. There was a strong Irish element within the organisation: its 1861 annual meeting was held in Dublin,[40] and Irish presidents of the MPA included Dr Lalor of the Richmond Lunatic Asylum (1861), Dr J.E. Duncan (1875), Dr Conolly Norman of Grangegorman Mental Hospital (1895), Dr W. R. Dawson (1911), Dr M.J. Nolan of Downpatrick (1924), Dr R. Leeper (1931) and Professor John Dunne (1955).[41]

English was an active MPA participant throughout her membership of the organisation. In July 1917, for example, the Summer Meeting of the Irish Division of the MPA was held in Ballinasloe 'by the kind invitation of Dr John Mills (Medical Superintendent)' and English was, of course, amongst the (small) attendance.[42]

English was also a member of the British Medical Association[43] but not the Royal College of Physicians of Ireland (which was not required in order to practice as a doctor). In any case, in addition to her career in medicine, English had a second passion to keep her busy: Irish nationalist politics.

Political Background

English grew up and lived during a uniquely eventful time in Irish history, as Ireland emerged from a lengthy period of British rule and steps were taken to establish an independent Irish Republic. From 1 January 1801 to 6 December 1922 Ireland formed part of the United Kingdom of Great Britain and Ireland, a situation which generated continual unrest among the Irish.[44] As a result, there were a succession of rebellions.

The struggle for Irish freedom took a new turn in the late 1870s, when English was a young child, as the Irish National Land League was founded in Castlebar, County Mayo on 21 October 1879. The Land League sought to support tenant farmers (predominantly Roman Catholic) in their conflicts with landlords (predominantly Protestant) regarding rent and land ownership. The organisation focused on achieving the 'three Fs' for tenants: fair rent, fixity of tenure and free sale. Its first president was Charles Stewart Parnell (1846–91), an Irish landlord and later founder of the Irish Parliamentary Party.

The establishment of the Land League was followed by a 'Land War', during which the Land League was declared illegal. With many of the men of the Land League in prison, the Ladies' Land League was founded in 1880 by Fanny Parnell and Anna Parnell, sisters of Charles Stewart Parnell. The Ladies' Land League aimed to continue the work of the men in prison, and by 1882 had 500 branches throughout Ireland. Many of its members would later join Cumann na mBan (Women's League),[45] in which English played a significant role.[46]

In parallel with the Land War, this period in Irish history also saw significant political developments in relation to self-government or 'home rule' for Ireland.

During the first decade of the twentieth century, Sinn Féin was established as a political party with the aim of achieving self-government for Ireland and a series of Home Rule Bills was presented to the House of Commons, seeking self-government.

Following both considerable political activity and considerable delay, a Home Rule Bill (the Government of Ireland Act) was duly passed in 1914 but did not come into force, owing to the occurrences of World War I and the Easter Rising.[47] Following the Rising, however, the government's execution of republican leaders deepened public sympathy for Ireland's republican cause, and Sinn Féin was victorious in the 1918 election, following which 'Dáil Éireann' (the Irish parliament) met in Dublin in January 1919.[48] Irish independence was declared and Éamon de Valera, an American-born Irish nationalist (and friend of English), was elected President of Dáil Éireann in April 1919.[49]

As the earlier stages of these events unfolded throughout the 1870s and 1880s, English was growing up in Mullingar, County Westmeath. Her childhood coincided with a period of particularly intense social and political unrest locally as 'the poverty gripping Ireland at the time of the famine led to mounting unrest [and] agrarian violence mounted in Mullingar... Agrarian and political violence remained very common in 1860s Westmeath. At least eighty homicides took place in the county between 1849 and 1870'.[50]

English was a young child during this 'Land War' but was undoubtedly aware of the political and social problems of the day: English's grandfather, Richard, was master of the Oldcastle Workhouse and the destitution that English witnessed others suffering while she was a child would have affected her.[51] This awareness contributed not only to English's political activism, but also her empathy with the marginalised and dispossessed, an empathy which was to define her working life for almost four decades at Ballinasloe District Asylum.

Personal and Family Life

English remained close to her family throughout her life, even though she spent almost four decades in Ballinasloe, County Galway, and was later buried there alongside her patients.[52] In 1911, for example, although she had been working in Ballinasloe since 1904, English was back in Mullingar on census night (2 April 1911), where she was recorded at 8 Earl Street as 'single' and a 'doctor of medicine'.[53]

English's father, now aged fifty-nine years, was also resident along with her sister, Lilian, aged thirty-one years, 'single' and a 'pharmaceutical chemist' (like their father).[54] Two others were present too: Alfred Hanrahan from County

Clare, a 'chemist assistant' aged twenty-four years, and Mary Davitt from County Westmeath, a 'general servant' aged seventeen years.

English's brother Jeremiah Pierce qualified with a Licentiate of Apothecaries' Hall of Ireland (LAH) (an alternative medical qualification) in Dublin on 19 September 1913.[55] Jeremiah Pierce registered as a doctor on 28 October 1913 and practiced in Castlerea, County Roscommon.[56] Jeremiah Pierce married Gertrude Mary J. Fitzgibbon in 1914 in Dublin and a son, Diarmuid Michael Francis, was born on 20 September 1915 in Castlerea. Diarmuid qualified in medicine (MB BCh) from the National University of Ireland in 1942 and registered as a doctor on 16 February 1942. By the following year Diarmuid was at the Ballinasloe asylum from which his aunt had just retired the previous year. Diarmuid later went to England, where he died in Sheffield, Yorkshire in March 1987.

Jeremiah Pierce's daughter, Nora Mary, was born on 28 December 1916 in Castlerea. She also qualified in medicine (MB BCh) from the National University of Ireland in 1942, the same year as her brother, Diarmuid. Nora registered as a doctor on 25 July 1942 and by the following year she too was at the Ballinasloe asylum with her brother. Like Diarmuid, Nora later went to England, to Birkenhead in Cheshire, and died in Kings Lynn, Norfolk in January 1996. Their father, Jeremiah Pierce, became medical officer to the Castlerea Union (workhouse) and died of pneumonia on 30 November 1921.[57] Following his death, Jeremiah's Pierce's widow and children went to live with English in her house on the grounds of the mental hospital in Ballinasloe.[58]

Another brother of English, Patrick Francis, became a bank official[59] and in 1901 was living in Ballybeg, Clareabbey, County Clare,[60] later moving to Howth, County Dublin.[61] He married in 1920 in Dublin. In 1944, the year of English's death, Patrick Francis had retired and was living in Blackrock, County Dublin. English died on 27 January 1944 without leaving a will so, on 17 July 1944, the High Court appointed Patrick Francis to administer her personal estate (see Chapter Five).[62] Clearly, English had retained links with her brother throughout her life, as examination of her estate revealed that she and Patrick Francis jointly held a £1000 3.25 per cent National Security Loan, valued at £1060 at the time of English's death.[63] Patrick Francis died in the Rathdown District of Dublin in 1949.

English's mother died in 1918 in Ballinasloe and her father died in 1925. As the census returns from 1901 and 1911 suggest, the English family home had benefitted from the security and stability of her father's occupation as a pharmacist and prominent position as a town commissioner. English herself clearly benefitted further from her position in a middle-class family as it afforded her opportunity to pursue secondary education, an increasingly common but still rare opportunity for a girl in 1880s Ireland. To counter-balance this relative privilege, the young English was inevitably aware of the suffering of her less fortunate countrymen, owing to her grandfather's position as master of the Oldcastle Workhouse nearby.

Her education at the Loreto Convent also likely played a role in shaping her outlook. As a Roman Catholic, religion played a significant role throughout English's life. During her long career in Ballinasloe, English attended mass in the Roman Catholic chapel at the mental hospital every Sunday. Liam Hanniffy, son of the assistant land steward at the hospital (John Hanniffy), recalls serving at mass there in the 1930s.[64] English would arrive at the chapel, wheeling her green bicycle and accompanied by her dogs: Victor, Isabel and Judy. Hanging from each handle-bar of her bicycle was a bag with cooked breakfasts for the priest and English: sausages, eggs and pudding, each in a carefully heated container.

Interestingly, English was not the only member of her family to achieve national distinction. Her cousin W.R.E. Murphy achieved distinction in the field of boxing when, as assistant Garda commissioner he founded the Garda Boxing Club and, in 1939, secured the European Boxing Championship for Dublin. Ireland won no fewer than three titles in that year and Murphy is duly celebrated as 'the father of Irish boxing'.[65]

Murphy's daughter, Joan, remembers meeting English on a number of occasions when Joan was a child aged between nine and twelve years, and English was in her fifties.[66] Joan remembers English as a tall, slim woman with twinkling eyes, who always made an impressive entrance. When she visited, English presented the children with books on Irish history. English was fond of Irish tweed and visited the fashion shops of Dublin requesting to see only Irish produce. Clearly, English made a deep impression on the Murphy children, and while English sometimes referred to her patients as her family, she remained deeply committed to her own family too, providing financial support for her nephews' education.

Like Murphy, English had a strong interest in sport, and this would later inform a significant part of her professional and personal life in Ballinasloe, as she promoted sport in the asylum and played golf herself (see Chapter Three). Her key interests, however, were improving the position of the mentally ill and contributing to the struggle for Irish independence (see Chapter Two).

In this context, English's relatively privileged childhood circumstances, combined with her strong character and intellectual ability, both heightened her social awareness and provided her with increased opportunity to effect change. She was especially concerned about Ireland's political situation: English was just eleven years of age when the Irish Government Bill 1886, which aimed to establish home rule in Ireland, was finally introduced, although it was defeated by thirty votes in the House of Commons.

As a result of this sequence of events, Ireland was still not self-governing or independent when English completed her medical education in 1903, and there seemed to be limited prospects for immediate progress. This was a situation that English was to work hard to rectify, and her prolonged commitment to the struggle for Irish freedom is considered next.

Notes

1. Birth Certificate, Adeline English, 10 January 1875 (General Register Office/ An tSeirbhís um Chlárú Sibhialta, Roscommon, Ireland); D. Kelly, *Between the Lines of History: People of Ballinasloe, Volume One* (Ballinasloe: Declan Kelly, 2000), p.24.
2. Marriage Certificate, Patrick English and Honora Mulvihill, 18 February 1873 (General Register Office/An tSeirbhís um Chlárú Sibhialta, Roscommon, Ireland).
3. Illingworth, Councillor Ruth, historian (interview in Mullingar, County Westmeath, 23 June 2013).
4. Kelly, *Between the Lines of History*, p.25.
5. I. Mulvany, 'The Intermediate Act and the education of girls', *Irish Educational Review*, 1 (October 1907), pp.14–20.
6. M. Ó hÓgartaigh, 'A quiet revolution: Irish women and second-level education, 1878–1930', *New Hibernia Review*, 13, 2 (Samhradh/Summer 2009), pp.36–51.
7. J. Harford, *The Opening of University Education to Women in Ireland* (Dublin: Irish Academic Press, 2007).
8. *Irish Press*, 28 January 1944; *Irish Times*, 29 January 1944; *East Galway Democrat*, 29 January 1944; Kelly, *Between the Lines of History*, p.25.
9. *Irish Press*, 28 January 1944. See also: *East Galway Democrat*, 29 January 1944.
10. F.O.C. Meenan, *Cecilia Street: The Catholic University School of Medicine, 1855–1931* (Dublin: Gill and Macmillan, 1987), p.2.
11. M. Ó hÓgartaigh, 'Women in university education in Ireland: the historical background', in A. Macdona (ed.), *From Newman to New Woman: UCD Women Remember* (Dublin: New Island Books, 2001), pp.iii–xi.
12. M. Ó hÓgartaigh, '"Is there any need of you?" Women in medicine in Ireland and Australia', *Australian Journal of Irish Studies*, 4 (2004), pp.162–71.
13. Meenan, *Cecilia Street*, p.7.
14. Ibid., p.38.
15. W. Rivington, *The Medical Profession* (Dublin: Fannin and Company, 1879), pp.135–7.
16. Meenan, *Cecilia Street*, p.82.
17. M. Ó hÓgartaigh, *Kathleen Lynn: Irishwoman, Patriot, Doctor* (Dublin: Irish Academic Press, 2006), p.12.
18. Meenan, *Cecilia Street*, p.83.
19. M.M. Macken, 'Women in the University and the College: a struggle within a struggle', in M. Tierney (ed.), *Struggle with Fortune: A Miscellany for the Centenary of the Catholic University of Ireland, 1854–1954* (Dublin: Browne and Nolan, 1954), p.151.

20. Census Return Forms for House Thirteen in Earls South Side (Mullingar Urban, Westmeath), 31 March 1901 (The National Archives of Ireland, Dublin).
21. Kelly, *Between the Lines of History*, p.25.
22. *St Stephen's* (college magazine of the Catholic University, Dublin), June 1903, p.266; Ó hÓgartaigh, *From Newman to New Woman*, pp.iii–xi.
23. *St Stephen's*, March 1902, p.93.
24. *St Stephen's*, February 1904, p.44.
25. Meenan, *Cecilia Street*, p.84.
26. *St Stephen's*, June 1904, p.89; M. Ó hÓgartaigh, *Quiet Revolutionaries: Irish Women in Education, Medicine and Sport, 1861–1964* (Dublin: The History Press Ireland, 2011), pp.193–4.
27. Ó hÓgartaigh, *From Newman to New Woman*, pp.iii–xi.
28. *Medical Directory for 1905* (London: J. & A. Churchill, 1905), p.1414; *Irish Press*, 28 January 1944; *East Galway Democrat*, 29 January 1944; *Irish Times*, 29 January 1944; F. Clarke, 'English, Adeline ('Ada')', in J. McGuire and J. Quinn (eds), *Dictionary of Irish Biography: From the Earliest Times to the Year 2002 (Volume 3, D-F)* (Cambridge: Royal Irish Academy and Cambridge University Press, 2009), pp.626–7.
29. *East Galway Democrat*, 29 January 1944; *Irish Press*, 28 January 1944; M. McNamara and P. Mooney, *Women in Parliament: 1918–2000* (Dublin: Wolfhound Press, 2000), p.79; F. Clarke, 'English, Adeline ('Ada')', in J. McGuire and J. Quinn (eds), *Dictionary of Irish Biography*, pp.626–7; L. Kelly, *Irish Women in Medicine, c.1880s–1920s: Origins, Education and Careers* (Manchester and New York: Manchester University Press, 2012), p.211.
30. Murray, J.P. *Galway: A Medico-Social History* (Galway: Kenny's Bookshop and Art Gallery, 1996), pp.195, 200.
31. Murray, *Galway*, p.198.
32. Meenan, *Cecilia Street*, p.85.
33. Personal communication, Francis Maunze, Archivist and Records Manager, Royal College of Psychiatrists, 17 Belgrave Square, London SW1X 8PG, England (3 April 2013).
34. Anonymous. 'Irish Division', *Journal of Mental Science*, 56, 235 (1910), p.776.
35. J. Reynolds, *Grangegorman: Psychiatric Care in Dublin since 1815* (Dublin: Institute of Public Administration in association with Eastern Health Board, 1992).
36. Anonymous, 'Irish Division', *Journal of Mental Science*, 63, 263 (1917), p.620.
37. T. Bewley, *Madness to Mental Illness: A History of the Royal College of Psychiatrists* (London: Royal College of Psychiatrists, 2008), p.10.
38. A. Collins, 'Eleonora Fleury captured', *British Journal of Psychiatry*, 203, 1 (2013), p.5; Bewley, *Madness to Mental Illness*, p.27.
39. *Medical Directory for 1905*, pp.1414, 1417.
40. Bewley, *Madness to Mental Illness*, p.20.
41. B.D. Kelly, 'Physical sciences and psychological medicine: the legacy of Prof John Dunne', *Irish Journal of Psychological Medicine*, 22, 2 (2005), pp.67–72. See also: Healy D. 'Irish psychiatry. Part 2: Use of the Medico-Psychological Association by its Irish members-plus ca change!', in G.E. Berrios and H. Freeman (eds), *150 Years of British Psychiatry, 1841–1991* (London: Gaskell/Royal College of Psychiatrists, 1991), pp.314–20.

42. Anonymous, 'Irish Division', *Journal of Mental Science*, 63, 263 (1917), p.620.

43. *Medical Directory for 1905*, p.1414.

44. F.S.L. Lyons, *Ireland Since the Famine* (London: Fontana, 1985).

45. C. McCarthy, *Cumann na mBan and the Irish Revolution* (Dublin: The Collins Press, 2007), pp.6–7.

46. *East Galway Democrat*, 29 January 1944.

47. McNamara and Mooney, *Women in Parliament: 1918–2000*, p.79; *Irish Press*, 28 January 1944; *East Galway Democrat*, 29 January 1944.

48. D. Ferriter, *The Transformation of Ireland 1900–2000* (London: Profile Books, 2004), pp.183–4.

49. Ferriter, *The Transformation of Ireland 1900–2000*, p.184; T.P. Coogan, *De Valera: Long Fellow, Long Shadow* (London: Hutchinson, 1993); D. Ferriter, *Judging Dev: A Reassessment of the Life and Legacy of Éamon de Valera* (Dublin: Royal Irish Academy, 2007).

50. R. Illingworth, *Mullingar: History and Guide* (Dublin: Nonsuch, 2007), pp.75, 84.

51. Kelly, *Between the Lines of History*, p.25.

52. *Irish Press*, 28 January 1944; *East Galway Democrat*, 29 January 1944.

53. Census Return Forms for House Eight in Earl Street (Mullingar South Urban, Westmeath), 2 April 1911 (The National Archives of Ireland, Dublin).

54. Census Return Forms for House Eight in Earl Street (Mullingar South Urban, Westmeath), 2 April 1911 (The National Archives of Ireland, Dublin). English was 'the younger daughter of the late PJ English and Mrs Nora English, Mullingar' (*Irish Times*, 29 January 1944).

55. Apothecaries' Hall of Ireland Roll of Licentiates (Commencing April 1913) (Royal College of Physicians of Ireland, Dublin, Ireland), p.1.

56. Kelly, *Between the Lines of History*, p.24.

57. *Irish Times*, 1 December 1921.

58. Hanniffy, Dr Liam, Assistant Inspector of Mental Hospitals (retired) and son of Mr John Hanniffy, assistant land steward, Mental Hospital, Ballinasloe, County Galway (interview in Portlaoise, County Laois, 27 May 2013).

59. Census Return Forms for House One in Ballybeg (Clareabbey, County Clare), 31 March 1901 (The National Archives of Ireland, Dublin).

60. Ibid.; Kelly, *Between the Lines of History*, p.24.

61. Census Return Forms for House Ninety-Eight in Burrow South (Howth, County Dublin), 2 April 1911 (The National Archives of Ireland, Dublin).

62. Grant of Administration (Adeline English) 17 July 1944 (National Archives, Bishop Street, Dublin, Ireland).

63. Schedule of Assets (Adeline English) 17 July 1944 (National Archives, Bishop Street, Dublin, Ireland).

64. Hanniffy, Dr Liam, Assistant Inspector of Mental Hospitals (retired) and son of Mr John Hanniffy, assistant land steward, Mental Hospital, Ballinasloe, County Galway (interview in Portlaoise, County Laois, 27 May 2013).

65. U. O'Connor, 'Let's honour the father of Irish boxing', *Sunday Independent*, 26 August 2012.

66. Murphy, Ms Joan Patricia, first cousin (once removed) of English (interview in Ballinasloe, Country Galway on 3 May 2013).

CHAPTER TWO

─────── ℘ ℭ ───────

Politics: Cumann na mBan, Easter Rising, War of Independence, Second Dáil and Civil War, 1914–29

Dr Ada English (National University) said that she was against the Treaty… If the oaths were omitted from the Treaty she could accept it under force, but while these oaths were in it, in which they were asked to accept the King of England as head of the Irish State and to accept the status of British subjects, they could not accept it… She denied that the country was in favour of the Treaty… It would be a complete spiritual surrender, and it would not bring peace but bitter division to the country. She was sorry to see unity in the Dáil broken up but she would be more sorry to see the unity that would accept the Treaty.

Irish Times, 5 January 1922.[1]

English lived during a uniquely eventful period of Irish history, as Ireland emerged from a lengthy period of British rule and steps were taken to establish an independent Irish Republic. English played an active role in these events, combining nationalist politics with medical work at Ballinasloe District Asylum over four tumultuous decades.

English, like many others, sought an independent Ireland. On this basis, she was politically active in the Irish Volunteers (1913) and Cumann na mBan (1914), and deeply involved in the War of Independence (1919–21), Second

19

Dáil (1921–2) and Civil War (1922–3). She was 'an intimate friend of Joseph McDonagh, Patrick Pearse, Arthur Griffith, Liam Mellows and very many other national figures of the struggle for independence'.[2] These organisations, events and personalities, and English's connections with them, are examined in this chapter.

Irish Volunteers (1913) and Cumann Na mBan (1914)

As the movement toward Irish independence grew in strength at the start of the twentieth century, English's interest in Irish language, heritage and nationalist politics grew in parallel. English was tutored in Irish language and poetry by Pádraig Pearse, an Irish poet, patriot and one of the leaders of the Easter Rising.[3] Pearse, an iconic figure in Irish history, had a broad range of involvements in Irish language, heritage and politics during this period. In 1899, for example, Father Delaney, president of the Jesuit University College, Dublin invited the Gaelic League to provide Irish classes to his students and Pearse became the teacher.[4] There were fewer than a dozen students in the class and Pearse is remembered as shy, earnest and studious. One member of that class, Louis J. Walsh, DJ (District Justice), later recalled their tuition by Pearse:

> It was, [Walsh] says, when he came to Dublin about 1899 to prepare for matriculation at old University College that he and other students got up a special class once a week and their teacher was the youthful P.H. Pearse, then still unknown outside a small circle of enthusiasts, and not yet editor of *An Claidheamh Soluis*. Among still surviving members of that class are Mr Walsh's sister, now Mrs Concannon, TD, and author of historical studies; Professor Merriman, Dr Ada English and Professor Mary Macken.[5]

Under Pearse's guidance,[6] English became a fluent Irish speaker.[7] Perhaps the most famous of Pearse's students at these classes was James Joyce, who later achieved fame as the author of *Ulysses* (1922) and *Finnegans Wake* (1939).[8] Joyce, however, found the Irish classes boring and was irritated by Pearse's habit of denigrating English in order to elevate Irish.[9] Joyce ultimately quit the classes in order to learn Norwegian, the language of Henrik Ibsen, the celebrated Norwegian playwright.

This was by no means the only time Joyce was to become disillusioned with his educational endeavours in Dublin: during the academic session 1903/1904, Joyce briefly attended lectures and visited the dissection room at the Catholic University School of Medicine on Cecilia Street, from which

English graduated in 1903.[10] Joyce had initially hoped to become a doctor but his enthusiasm waned when he was exposed to chemistry, a subject in which he could generate no interest.

Notwithstanding Joyce's disapproval, Pearse's classes in 1899 were popular and continued for another year.[11] Pearse went on, in 1908, to found St Enda's School (Scoil Éanna) in Rathfarnham, County Dublin, where pupils were taught in both Irish and English languages. The school ran into financial trouble, however, and supporters were invited to buy shares in order to shore up its finances. English purchased £5 worth of shares on 22 January 1912 but by the middle of 1912 Scoil Éanna Ltd was in liquidation and investors only received six pence in respect of each £1 invested.[12]

St Enda's remained, nonetheless, a significant location for Irish nationalists and it was there that, in 1915, the uniform of Cumann na mBan was worn in public for the first time.[13] By that time, it was apparent that English was not only interested in Irish language and culture, but also deeply committed to the Irish nationalist struggle. To this end, she joined both the Irish Volunteers and Cumann na mBan.[14]

The Irish Volunteers (Óglaigh na hÉireann) was founded in Dublin on 25 November 1913.[15] It was a military organisation with the explicit aim of promoting home rule for Ireland, in opposition to the Ulster Volunteers. The central aim of the Irish Volunteers was 'to secure and maintain the rights and liberties common to the whole people of Ireland'.[16] The organisation was prepared to use military force to defend these 'rights and liberties' if necessary. Eoin MacNeill, an Irish scholar and nationalist, was a key figure in the establishment of the Volunteers and became its chief-of-staff. English was a medical officer with the organisation.[17]

Despite widespread support for the new organisation amongst both men and women, the precise position of women within the Volunteers was unclear. Its manifesto stated:

> Volunteers will be enabled to aid the Volunteer forces in various capacities. There will also be work for the women to do, and there are signs that the women of Ireland, true to their record, are especially enthusiastic for the success of the Volunteers. We propose for the Volunteer organisation the widest possible base.[18]

This passage is unclear about the extent to which women were to be involved, and what, precisely, their roles might be. Against this background, a female wing of the Irish Volunteers, called Cumann na mBan (Women's League), was founded in 1914. The inaugural meeting of Cumann na mBan was held at Wynn's Hotel,

Dublin on 2 April 1914.[19] The constitution of the new organisation outlined its aims as follows:

1. To advance the cause of Irish Liberty.
2. To organise Irish women in furtherance of this object.
3. To assist in arming and equipping a body of Irishmen for the defence of Ireland.
4. To form a fund for these purposes to be called the 'Defence of Ireland Fund'.[20]

The manifesto of Irish Volunteers had stated that volunteers would 'be enrolled according to the district in which they live'.[21] Cumann na mBan recruited along similar lines. English, ever-enthusiastic for the cause, was a founder member of the Cumann na mBan branch in Ballinasloe and subsequently an executive member of the national organisation.[22] A branch of Cumann na mBan was set up in the asylum in Ballinasloe with English as chairperson.[23]

From the outset, Cumann na mBan was the subject of considerable criticism and debate. Hanna Sheehy Skeffington, for example, an Irish suffragette and nationalist, publicly bemoaned Cumann na mBan's focus on providing arms for the men of the Volunteers and its alleged failure to work for greater equality between men and women.[24] Regardless, six months after its inaugural meeting Cumann na mBan had over sixty branches throughout Ireland. At the Cumann na mBan convention in Dublin in October 1915 the organisation unanimously elected its first president, Jennie Wyse Power, an Irish feminist, nationalist and founder member of Sinn Féin.[25]

Easter Rising (1916)

Against this backdrop of nationalist organisation and activity, an Irish republican uprising against British rule took place in Easter week, 1916. In essence, the rebels sought to establish an Irish Republic. The Rising was largely organised by the Irish Republican Brotherhood which had been founded in the 1850s with the aim of achieving an independent democratic republic in Ireland. To this end, members of the Irish Volunteers, Irish Citizen Army and Cumann na mBan seized control of key locations in Dublin at Easter 1916. An Irish republic was declared and a provisional government established at the General Post Office on Sackville Street (later O'Connell Street) in Dublin's city centre.

The Rising which had been scheduled for Easter Sunday did not commence until Easter Monday, leading to considerable confusion amongst potential participants. Some potential participants, including members of

Cumann na mBan, had expected 'manoeuvres' rather than an uprising on Easter Sunday.[26] When military activity finally commenced on Easter Monday, public uncertainty about unfolding events meant there was an insufficient groundswell of support for the rebels amongst the general Irish population. The rebels were, in any case, no military match for British forces, and the Rising was crushed relatively quickly. Pádraig Pearse and fourteen other leaders, including Pearse's brother Willie, were court-martialled and executed by firing squad. Roger Casement, an Irish Nationalist and poet, was hanged at Pentonville Prison in England.

A lack of co-ordination surrounded the Rising, but military activity was not confined to Dublin. In Ashbourne, County Meath, there was a substantial attack on a Royal Irish Constabulary Barracks. In Cork, 1,200 volunteers assembled, under the command of Tomás Mac Curtain, although they did not engage in action owing to a misinterpretation of their orders. In Wexford, one hundred volunteers took over the town of Enniscorthy for three days, before British reinforcements were dispatched; rebel leaders were escorted to Arbour Hill Prison in Dublin and ordered by Pearse to surrender.

There was also significant military action in County Galway, where English was active in both the Irish Volunteers and Cumann na mBan. The uprising in Galway was led by Liam Mellows, an Irish nationalist and Sinn Féin politician.[27] Mellows was born in Manchester, England and grew up in County Wexford. He was heavily influenced by Thomas Clarke, an Irish revolutionary leader later executed after the Easter Rising. In his formative years, Mellows was also affected by the socialism of James Connolly, another Irish republican leader executed after the Rising. Mellows had met Connolly at the home of Constance Markievicz, a celebrated nationalist, socialist and suffragette who became the first woman elected to the British House of Commons in 1918 (see below).[28]

Mellows's involvement in Irish nationalism resulted in his imprisonment by the British on several occasions. Following an escape from Reading jail in England, Mellows fled to the west of Ireland where he orchestrated the military activity during the Easter Rising. During Easter week, Mellows led a force of 700 Irish Volunteers who engaged in military action at several locations throughout County Galway. In Clarinbridge and Oranmore, the rebels attacked two police stations. In Carnmore, two members of the Royal Irish Constabulary were killed.

Members of Cumann na mBan played a more prominent role in the 1916 Rising in Galway than they did elsewhere.[29] In Dublin, there was particularly deep confusion about the role of Cumann na mBan during Easter week: de Valera, for example, led a group of rebels at Boland's Mills but appears to have sent word to members of Cumann na mBan assembled in Merrion Square that they were not needed and could return home.[30] In Galway, by contrast, fifteen to twenty members of Cumann na mBan served actively with Mellows.[31]

Given that English had joined both the Irish Volunteers[32] and Cumann na mBan,[33] was a friend of Mellows[34] and worked in nearby Ballinasloe, it is little surprise that she is reported to have served as medical officer for the wounded rebels.[35] Moreover, while members of Cumann na mBan at most other locations were engaged primarily in dispatch work and various other tasks,[36] members of Cumann na mBan in Galway with Mellows played significant roles in important military decisions, including presenting their views during discussions about possible surrender.[37]

Mellows's forces were, however, very poorly armed, with only 300 shotguns and twenty-five rifles. They also ran short of food and, to add to their woes, a British cruiser, HMS *Gloucester*, arrived in Galway Bay and began to shell the fields around Athenry where the rebels were based. As a result, the rebels dispersed and many were arrested. Mellows was amongst those who escaped and he went to the United States, where he was quickly arrested for allegedly aiding the German side during the World War I. Nonetheless, in the 1918 general election, Mellows was elected as a Sinn Féin member of the First Dáil and later worked with the Irish Republican Army during the War of Independence, was elected (with English) to the Second Dáil, and became deeply involved (like English) in the Civil War.

Following the Easter Rising, English continued her work in the asylum in Ballinasloe, just a few miles from the fields of Athenry, the scene of so much military activity in 1916. The Rising was undoubtedly a major event in English's life. It not only represented a dramatic attempt to realize the nationalist ideals in which she believed so strongly, but was also significant and quite possibly traumatic on a personal level. English was, as her *Irish Times* obituary highlighted, 'an intimate friend of Joseph McDonagh, Patrick Pearse, Arthur Griffith and Liam Mellows'.[38] While Mellows survived the 1916 Rising, some of English's other friends did not; most notably Pearse, who was executed in its aftermath, leading to considerable public outcry.

Later, English was to experience many more personal losses in the cause of Irish nationalism.[39] Joseph MacDonagh another Sinn Féin politician, would later die on hunger strike during the Civil War. George Clancy, republican mayor of Limerick, another friend of English, was shot by British forces in 1921, during the War of Independence.[40] Even more tragically, Mellows was eventually executed by his own countrymen in 1922.[41] These losses of so many friends and comrades must have weighed heavily on English, but do not appear to have diminished her life-long commitment to Irish nationalism.

War of Independence (1919–21)

The decade following the 1916 Easter Rising was a period of continued political strife in Ireland with the advent of a War of Independence with Great Britain, followed by the proposal of the divisive Anglo-Irish Treaty and a bitter Civil War.

In the immediate aftermath of the Rising, on 8 May 1916, the majority of the seventy-seven women who had been imprisoned during hostilities, many of whom were members of Cumann na mBan, were released from prison.[42] A minority, including Dr Kathleen Lynn, Madeline ffrench-Mullen (see Chapter Four) and Mary MacSwiney (see below), were detained for longer periods, but all were released by Christmas 1916, with one notable exception: Constance Markievicz.[43]

Markievicz was initially sentenced to death for her part in the Rising, but this was later commuted to life imprisonment apparently owing to her gender.[44] Markievicz was released in 1917 as part of the British government's general amnesty for those who took part in the Rising. She went on to become the first woman elected to the British House of Commons in 1918 but, along with seventy-two other Sinn Féin representatives, refused to take up her seat. In 1919, Markievicz was in Holloway prison in England when the First Dáil assembled in Dublin and an Irish Republic was declared. Like English, Markievicz was elected to the Second Dáil in 1921 and went on to play an active role in the Civil War.

The period between the 1916 Easter Rising and War of Independence was also a time of intensive political activity for English. The file the British Army kept on English records that she was 'present at a Sinn Féin meeting in Galway Town' on 1 January 1918.[45] On 3 March 1918 she 'was reported to be president of the local Cumann na mBan, which she organised'. On 9 June 1918 she 'took a prominent part in the women's anti-conscription demonstration at Ballinasloe … and was chief organiser'. Cumann na mBan had a long history of opposition to conscription to the British Army.[46]

Given this level of sustained engagement and political activism, it is little surprise that English became involved in the War of Independence. The War of Independence was waged primarily by the Irish Republican Army (IRA) against British forces in Ireland. The IRA had emerged from the Irish Volunteers following their defeat in 1916. The organisation was established at a convention in Dublin on 27 October 1917 and English had many close links with its early leaders.

Éamon de Valera, for example, was elected first president of the IRA at the 1917 convention.[47] English, a close friend of de Valera,[48] reportedly helped him and various others hide out at the asylum in Ballinasloe.[49] In the Second Dáil,

English provided strong support for de Valera for the position of President of the Irish Republic in 1921.

Also at the 1917 IRA convention, Cathal Brugha, an Irish revolutionary politician, became Chairman of the Resident Executive of the IRA. It is reported that English later served alongside Brugha at the Hammam Hotel in Dublin during the Civil War.[50] Austin Stack, an Irish revolutionary and politician, was also elected to the IRA national executive at the 1917 convention and later offered English the position of Resident Medical Superintendent of Sligo Mental Hospital. English declined, refusing to be separated from her patients in Ballinasloe.[51]

Two years after the 1917 IRA convention, on the same day the First Dáil convened at the Mansion House in Dublin, members of the IRA shot two Royal Irish Constabulary (RIC) officers in County Tipperary. While this was by no means the first act of violence since 1916, it marked an intensification of violence against British forces, with particular focus on members of the RIC, the British police force in Ireland. As the War of Independence developed, a policy of ostracism of RIC members was put in place, with the result that recruitment to the RIC fell sharply and the rate of resignations rose. English was no stranger to problems with the RIC: on one occasion, members of the RIC physically removed her from a chair upon which she was standing to speak, and ejected her from Ballinasloe Town Hall.[52]

Cumann na mBan also remained active during the War of Independence, often working with the IRA in specific military actions against the British (such as ambushes) as well as transporting weapons and assisting with intelligence gathering.[53] English played an active role as a member of the Executive of Cumann na mBan during this period.[54] The British Army file on English also noted that English's 'name appears in secret documents seized from Michael Collins as the delegate from Co Galway to the Annual Convention of Cumann na mBan, 1919–1920'.[55]

As the War of Independence progressed, the British government sent two paramilitary police forces to assist the RIC in Ireland: the Black and Tans and the Auxiliaries. Violence intensified further in late 1920, and by July 1921 the armed conflict appeared to have reached a state of stalemate. There was considerable disenchantment with the persistent violence on both sides and a truce was agreed on 11 July 1921. This led to further negotiations and the emergence of the Anglo-Irish Treaty which, in turn, precipitated the Civil War.[56]

Throughout War of Independence, English worked constantly at the Ballinasloe District Asylum, a large institution with almost 2,000 patients and several hundred staff members. English's position at the asylum offered her a unique opportunity to help undermine the RIC, as she used offers of jobs at the asylum to persuade members of the RIC members to leave the force. For example, Laurence Garvey, a lieutenant with the Athenry Company of the Irish Volunteers, provided a Witness Statement to the Bureau of Military History in which he outlined his efforts to induce an RIC member named Curley ('a native of Clontuskert') to resign:

> Curley resigned from the RIC. He signed some papers which Seamus Hogan, now Professor in Cork University, presented to him and he got a job in Ballinasloe Mental Hospital through Dr Ada English. As far as I remember, Dr English arranged jobs in the Mental Hospital for any RIC man who could be induced to resign.[57]

Throughout the War of Independence, English also continued her involvement with Sinn Féin and Cumann na mBan. On 19 January 1921, however, she was dramatically arrested in Ballinasloe. The *Irish Times* reported the events of the day in some detail:

> Following a visit to her house on Tuesday, Dr Ada English, assistant resident medical superintendent of the Ballinasloe District Asylum, was arrested on Wednesday morning at 8 o'clock. She was conveyed under a strong escort of police and military to Galway jail by motor lorry at 11 o'clock. Dr English is a prominent Sinn Féiner and Gaelic Leaguer.[58]

On 22 January 1921 the *Western News and Galway Leader* reported English's arrest as 'the most serious news item in this district'.[59] They noted that English was arrested at the asylum where 'her quarters were raided' and 'she was arrested, it is believed, in consequence of papers found in her possession'.

English was not the only republican woman arrested in Galway that day: Alice Cashel, another member of Cumann na mBan and Sinn Féin activist, was also detained.[60] In 1920, Cashel had been elected as a Sinn Féin member of Galway County Council and was Vice-Chairman of the Council from 1920 to 1921. Unlike English, Cashel later provided a Witness Statement to the Bureau of Military History, in which she described her arrest in 1921 and her experiences while in custody:

> On my way to the Council Offices I was arrested and brought into Eglinton Street Police Barracks. I was brought upstairs and from a window I could see the Councillors and Rate Collectors making their way to meeting. Later I heard that they too were arrested for the day and that no meeting was held. Still looking out of my window, I saw a lorry of Auxillaries go down the street and with them in the lorry was a fashionably dressed

woman whom I took to be one of their wives. I was shocked at her assurance. But the lorry came back, with the lady still in it, and stopped at the barracks. In a few minutes the door of my room was opened and the lady was ushered in – no wife of an Auxiliary but a prisoner. She was Dr Ada English who had been arrested that morning at Ballinasloe.[61]

The two high–profile prisoners were soon moved from the Eglinton Street Police Barracks:

> They then evidently decided to bring us before the military authorities at Renmore. After a short time we were ordered out to a waiting car and under police escort we were driven off to Renmore Barracks. Even there there was delay in receiving us. I remember one fat policeman of our escort grumbling as we waited: 'It's all right for you – you will get all the glory and I'll get all the blame.' At last we were brought inside to be interviewed. An oily suave, half–police, half–soldier interviewed us separately … He was most polite to me so much so that when I went out I said to Dr English and my fat escort: 'I think I am going home.' 'If you call jail home,' said the fat one, 'you're going home.'[62]

Ironically, Renmore Barracks in Galway, where Cashel and English were interviewed by the 'oily suave, half–police, half–soldier', was later re–named Mellows Barracks (Dún Úi Maoilíosa) in honour of Liam Mellows, the nationalist rebel who served in 1916[63] and would later be executed during the Civil War.[64]

Following their interview in Renmore Barracks on 19 January 1921, English and Cashel were taken back to Galway Jail, located where the Cathedral of Our Lady Assumed into Heaven and Saint Nicholas, Galway stands today. Prison records state that English was 168 centimetres in height and weighed fifty–nine kilograms, with brown hair, grey eyes, a 'fresh' complexion and 'false upper teeth'.[65] Cashel was 170 centimetres in height and weighed seventy–two kilograms, with brown hair, blue eyes, a 'fresh' complexion and a 'birth mark on [her] right cheek'. English was an 'assistant medical officer, Ballinasloe Asylum' whereas Cashel was of 'independent means'. Both were unmarried and Roman Catholic in religion.

According to Cashel, conditions in the prison were difficult, although not impossibly so:

> This was my second time in this jail and on the question of our cells being raised, I looked around and chose one with a broken window – and it was January! – as I remembered feeling stifled when I was there last April. If

the window was broken I could rest assured that I would have air. We were given plank beds with mattresses and bed clothes, and on these we slept for some weeks until a humane army inspector arrived and was shocked at our condition. He ordered proper beds – a luxury which we could now appreciate.[66]

Cashel's niece, Patricia Lavelle later recalled when she and other family members visited Cashel:

We all went to visit [Alice Cashel] in jail. We found her in good company having Dr Ada English and Anita McMahon from Achill as her fellow prisoners. We brought her books and the makings of a hand-tufted hearth rug, and an extra pillow and a hot water bottle. She was in prison for most of that spring, but the Governor of the prison treated the three militant ladies with as much consideration as they themselves would allow, and we believed that they took an intellectual enjoyment out of arguing the toss of their political animosity whenever they came across him. This broke the tedium of prison life. We were sad as we left the prison and knew that she remained there under lock and key, but we were proud of her – an aunt important enough to be in prison.[67]

On 24 February 1921, English and Cashel were tried by 'Field General Court Martial' in Galway.[68] English was sentenced to 'nine months imprisonment without hard labour' for 'having a document relating to an unlawful association'.[69] As the *Irish Times* reported, English had been found in possession of 'a considerable quantity of seditious literature … including papers relating to the Cumann na mBan, details of activities, and Dáil Eireann Convention'.[70]

Cashel was sentenced to 'six months without hard labour' for 'having documents intended to cause disaffection'.[71] In her Witness Statement to the Bureau of Military History, Cashel provided a characteristically colourful version of events:

After six weeks we were summoned before a Field General Courtmartial, in Renmore Barracks – a most formal, pompous affair, members sworn in, etc., and all to no purpose, as we would not recognise the Court. As to the charges against me, I said that I was carrying out the instructions of the only Government I recognised. Well, I was sentenced to six months imprisonment and Dr English, against whom the charges were her activities in Cumann na mBan, to nine months. We were then taken back to jail.[72]

The *Western News and Galway Leader* also reported on the court martial:

> Both [English and Cashel] were charged with having documents relating
> to Cumann na mBan. The ladies objected to the court but were found
> guilty... They were removed to Galway prison by private motor. Dr
> English objected to the court on the ground that its members 'were in
> the pay of the enemy'. Some of them, would, no doubt, be glad to have
> half Dr English's pay from the same enemy.[73]

English and Cashel were two of approximately fifty women imprisoned in 1921.
Many were untried. Some were just fined.[74] Others, like English and Cashel,
received sentences which varied between three days and life imprisonment.[75]
Interestingly, Cashel was not the only high-profile woman imprisoned alongside
English in Galway jail at this time: Geraldine Plunkett Dillon, a prominent
republican activist, sister of Joseph Plunkett and wife of Professor Thomas
Dillon, was also there.[76] In her memoir, Dillon wrote about her time in prison
with English:

> It was beautifully quiet in the jail but it was the usual mess and very dirty.
> I was wakened in the middle of the night being bitten by such vermin
> as I have never seen before or since for size and variety, which were only
> got rid of by several disinfectant baths. Eight Galway county councillors
> had been arrested a few months before; Alice Cashel, the vice-chairman,
> was court-martialled and sentenced to six months for having documents
> and Dr Ada English of the mental hospital got nine months. They were
> great people and both in the so-called hospital of the jail; Dr English
> had got some kind of food poisoning and Miss Cashel was nursing her,
> the usual prison arrangement. My friend Bid McHugh sent in a dinner
> each day for me until, after three days, I was put in the hospital and spent
> my time cooking for Dr English, Alice Cashel and myself, which I really
> enjoyed. I cooked the prison rations which they had requested to be sent
> in raw, but there was not enough food for any length of time and it was
> quite mad. A lump of meat, four black potatoes, a piece of dirty bread
> and margarine, milk, but no vegetables. I cooked at the open fire in the
> hospital room in a frying pan and a smuggled saucepan and made bread
> puddings in a cake tin. The only other woman political prisoner was Miss
> Anita MacMahon from Westport, who did not mix with the rest of us
> except for an occasional hour of Bridge. Except for certain times when
> the prison spy was expected, the doors were not locked and there were
> little or no regulations. The prison doctor, Dr Kincaid, was a loyalist and

a savage. He used to inspect the hospital very early in the morning but never came back except once, when he reported the hospital as dirty for three crumbs on a floor and the medical inspector arrived from Dublin. He just chatted to Dr English for an hour about mental illnesses and went away laughing.[77]

English served just part of her nine-month sentence, before her sentence was commuted on 15 May 1921[78] and she was released owing to an episode of ptomaine poisoning (a form of food poisoning).[79] The following month, the *Western News and Galway Leader* reported that English 'has been released from imprisonment as a Sinn Féin offender on health grounds and recuperating in the south of France'.[80]

The British Army file on English records that she was 'released from Galway prison [on the] 13-5-21 on grounds of ill-health and on giving an undertaking to reside outside Counties Galway and Mayo'.[81] A subsequent note records that 'although not residing in Ballinasloe since her release, it is believed she has been active in connection with the Sinn Féin movement'. Indeed English was: in May 1921, while in prison, English was elected unopposed to Dáil Éireann, as a Sinn Féin candidate for the National University of Ireland constituency.[82]

Second Dáil (1921–2)

Sinn Féin had been established on 28 November 1905 with the aim 'to establish in Ireland's capital a national legislature endowed with the moral authority of the Irish nation'.[83] The party was founded by Arthur Griffith, an Irish writer and politician, who would later serve as President of Dáil Éireann from 10 January to 12 August 1922.

From the outset, Sinn Féin welcomed female members. As early as 1907, its national executive included several women, including Jennie Wyse Power and Mary Murphy. English was a close friend of Griffith[84] and member of the East Galway Comhairle Ceanntair of Sinn Féin,[85] having joined the Ballinasloe branch on its foundation in 1910.[86] She was also an active member of Cumann na mBan.[87]

In the 1918 general election, Sinn Féin won seventy-three of Ireland's 105 seats in the British House of Commons in 1918 but the seventy-three Sinn Féin representatives, including Markievicz, refused to take up their seats. Instead, they assembled in Dublin and proclaimed Dáil Éireann, the parliament of Ireland. The first meeting of Dáil Éireann (the First Dáil) took place at the Mansion House in Dublin on 21 January 1919. Cathal Brugha was elected as Ceann Comhairle (chairman) and an Irish republic declared.

Dáil Éireann was declared illegal by the British government but still met on a number of occasions at various locations. In December 1920, the British government passed the Government of Ireland Act, partitioning Ireland into two parts, each of which was to have a separate home-rule parliament: the House of Commons of Northern Ireland and the House of Commons of Southern Ireland. The First Dáil sat for the final time on 10 May 1921 ahead of these elections, in which English was elected to the Second Dáil.

Sinn Féin participated in the elections to both the House of Commons of Northern Ireland and the House of Commons of Southern Ireland. Sinn Féin did not, however, recognise these new parliaments and viewed the elections as elections to a 'Second Dáil' for all of the island of Ireland. The elections to the House of Commons of Northern Ireland took place on 24 May 1921. Sinn Féin won six seats out of fifty-two, while forty seats went to Unionists (supporting British rule) and six went to moderate nationalists. In the South, all candidates were returned unopposed: 124 Sinn Féin candidates and four independent Unionists, representing the University of Dublin (Trinity College).

As only Sinn Féin candidates recognised the Second Dáil, and five of these had been elected in both North and South, the Second Dáil, which convened from 16 August 1921 to 8 June 1922, comprised 125 members. One of these was English, who was elected unopposed for the National University of Ireland constituency.[88] The following year, during the Dáil debate on the Anglo-Irish Treaty, English commented:

> When I was selected as Deputy in this place I was very much surprised and, after I got out of jail, when I was well enough to see some of my constituents, I asked them how it came they selected me, and they told me they wanted someone they could depend on to stand fast by the Republic, and who would not let Galway down… *(cheers)*. That is what my constituents told me they wanted when they sent me here, and they have got it *(cheers)*.[89]

English was one of six Sinn Féin women elected to the Second Dáil; the others were Mary MacSwiney (see below), Constance Markievicz (see above), Margaret Pearse (mother of Padraig and Willie), Kate O'Callaghan (member of Cumann na mBan and an academic) and Kathleen Clarke (founder member of Cumann na mBan and first female Lord Mayor of Dublin, 1939-41).[90]

The Second Dáil was supportive of the truce in the War of Independence, which was agreed on 11 July 1921. While the truce helped to diminish hostilities at national level, it did not diminish English's republican activism: the British

Army file on English, in a section headed 'Activities Since The Truce' (undated), notes that 'after making a "blood and thunder" speech at Ballinasloe, she proceeded openly to enlist members of Cumann na mBan'.[91]

As a result of the truce, the Dáil, of which English was now part, could meet openly without fear of persecution, for the first time since 1919. Since April 1919, Éamon de Valera (Sinn Féin) had been 'President of Dáil Éireann' and one of the actions of the Second Dáil was to replace his position with another, titled 'President of the Irish Republic'. The purpose of this change was to have a 'Head of State' for Ireland and thus hopefully strengthen the Irish position in peace negotiations with Britain. In 1921, de Valera was duly nominated for the position of President of the Irish Republic by Sean MacEoin, a politician, soldier and, like English, Sinn Féin member of the Second Dáil.

In the Dáil debate on 26 August 1921, English strongly supported de Valera's nomination:

> I have very great pleasure in supporting the resolution put before you by Commandant MacEoin. There is no necessity for me to praise Éamon de Valera to the men and women of the Dáil or to the men and women of Ireland. He has been tested in times of the greatest stress both as a soldier and statesman. We all know how he has come out of it – and the enemy knows it. The fact that for the past forty years the enemy has refused Home Rule and now are offering most cheerfully what they called 'Dominion Status,' shows what has been done by him. As a new member of the Dáil, I should like to say how much we appreciate him and how much we are impressed by him. His desire for the fullest criticism, and his openness to any suggestions and readiness to accept them if they are any good; his courage and manifest honesty in placing before us everything which he is recommending to us, leaves us, even the dullest of us, under no delusion as to what we are asked to do. I have very much pleasure in supporting the motion.[92]

De Valera was duly elected President of the Irish Republic and the Dáil nominated *envoys plenipotentiary* for negotiations with Great Britain. These envoys included Arthur Griffith, a friend of English,[93] and Michael Collins, a Cork-born Irish revolutionary leader and participant in the 1916 Easter Rising. Collins had been a Sinn Féin member of the First Dáil and was, like English, a Sinn Féin member of the Second Dáil. He was appointed Minister for Finance in 1919.[94] As an *envoy plenipotentiary*, Collins played a key role in negotiating the Anglo-Irish Treaty in London during the autumn and winter of 1921.

This period also saw considerable debate and political activity in Ireland. On 21 September 1921, for example, the *Gloucester Citizen* reported on a 'Sinn Féin demonstration at Mullingar', where English had grown up:

> Enthusiastic scenes marked the visit of Commandant McKeon, Mrs Pearse, Mrs Thomas Clarke, Dr Ada English and other officials to Mullingar on Tuesday night. Large crowds took part in a great demonstration. Commandant McKeon in a stirring speech exhorted all young men to join the Irish Republican Army.[95]

The Treaty was signed by the envoys on 6 December 1921 and officially known as *Articles of Agreement for a Treaty Between Great Britain and Ireland*. The Treaty specified that an Irish Free State would be established within a year, as a self-governing dominion within the 'British Commonwealth of Nations'. It also provided for the withdrawal of British forces from most of Ireland and gave Northern Ireland the option of opting out of the Irish Free State (which it did). The Treaty stated that members of the Irish Free State parliament would have to take an oath of allegiance to the Irish Free State and swear to 'be faithful to His Majesty King George V, his heirs and successors by law, in virtue of the common citizenship'.

The Treaty had to be ratified both by the British Parliament (which occurred on 16 December 1921) and, in the words of the Treaty, by 'a meeting summoned for the purpose [of approving the Treaty] of the members elected to sit in the House of Commons of Southern Ireland'. The Second Dáil debated the Treaty for nine days, before voting on the matter on 7 January 1922. English strongly and publicly opposed the Treaty during the Dáil debate:

> I credit the supporters of the Treaty with being as honest as I am, but I have a sound objection to it. I think it is wrong; I have various reasons for objecting to it, but the main one is that, in my opinion, it was wrong against Ireland and a sin against Ireland ... while those oaths are in it, oaths in which we are asked to accept the King of England as head of the Irish State, and we are asked to accept the status of British citizens – British subjects – that we cannot accept. As far as I see the whole fight in this country for centuries has centred round that very point. We are now asked not only to acknowledge the King of England's claim to be King of Ireland, but we are asked to swear allegiance and fidelity ('No! No!') in virtue of that claim... The country wants no peace which gives away the independence of Ireland and destroys the Republic which has been established by the will of the Irish people... We repudiate the Republic if

this Treaty is passed; we repudiate it absolutely. It is a complete surrender and we don't get peace by it, but we get the certainty of a bitter split and division in this country…[96]

English, like many other participants in the Dáil debate, wished to invoke the memory of those who had died in the fight for Irish freedom. To articulate this, English and the other five women members of the Dáil – all of whom rejected the Treaty[97] – wore black attire throughout the Treaty debate.[98] Unlike most of her female colleagues in the Dáil, however, English had not personally experienced family bereavement, and was at pains to emphasise that her opposition to the Treaty was not based solely on personal bereavements:[99]

> There is a point I want to make. I think that it was a most brave thing today to listen to the speech by the deputy from Sligo [Alexander McCabe] in reference to the women members of An Dáil, claiming that they only have the opinions they have because they have a grievance against England, or because their men folk were killed and murdered by England's representatives in this country. It was a most unworthy thing for any man to say here. I can say this more freely because, I thank my God, I have no dead men to throw in my teeth as a reason for holding the opinions I hold. I should like to say that I think it most unfair to the women Teachtaí because Miss MacSwiney had suffered at England's hands. That, a Chinn Chomhairle, is really all I want to say. I am against the Treaty, and I am very sorry to be in opposition to *(nodding towards Mr Griffith and Mr Collins). (Cheers).*[100]

The following day, the *Irish Times* reported that English saw the treaty as 'a complete spiritual surrender, and it would not bring peace but bitter division to the country. She was sorry to see unity in the Dáil broken up but she would be more sorry to see the unity that would accept the Treaty'.[101] The historical context of English's remarks was clear, as reported in the *Irish Times*:

> For seven hundred years the Irish people had denied the right of England's kings in this country [Ireland], and they were now asked not only to acknowledge the claims of the King of England as head of Ireland, but they were also to acknowledge themselves as British subjects. It seemed to her [English] that the taking of these oaths was a complete surrender of Ireland's claim; that it was giving up the independence of their country. That was the main reason why she objected to the Treaty. She denied that the country was in favour of the Treaty. The country wanted peace, a peace that would be a real peace, a peace based on honour and friendship.[102]

As English's contributions suggest, the Dáil debate on the Treaty was heated and acrimonious. Nonetheless, the Dáil ratified the Treaty on 7 January 1922, with sixty-four members voting in favour, and fifty-seven (including English) against. English, like many others, foresaw trouble, pointing out that 'if this Treaty were accepted, and the Free State Government were in power, they would have to use the army if they wanted to keep the Treaty, to support the Treaty and this, she considered, meant England holding Ireland'.[103]

De Valera, who opposed the Treaty, resigned as president and Arthur Griffith, who supported it, was elected in his place on 9 January 1922.[104] Since the Treaty had to be ratified by the House of Commons of Southern Ireland too, the pro-Treaty members of the Dáil ended their boycott of the House of Commons of Southern Ireland and, along with its four Unionist members, ratified the Treaty in the House of Commons of Southern Ireland on 14 January 1922. Michael Collins, who supported the Treaty, was nominated as Chairman of the Provisional Government.

One of the terms of the Treaty was that the House of Commons of Southern Ireland and Second Dáil would be replaced by a single parliament for the Free State, so elections for the Third Dáil were held on 16 June 1922. English ran for the National University panel, having been 'proposed by A.E. Cleary, LLD [and] seconded by Thomas Derrig'.[105]

At national level, pro-Treaty Sinn Féin, led by Collins, won fifty-eight out of 128 seats, while anti-Treaty Sinn Féin, led by de Valera, won just thirty-six seats. Overall, pro-Treaty candidates (including pro-Treaty Sinn Féin candidates) won over 75 per cent of the vote and English was one of the anti-Treaty candidates not re-elected.[106]

More specifically, in the National University constituency English 'went out with 334 votes, being 194 short of the quota of 528'.[107] As a result, in the words of the *New York Times*, 'Dr Ada English, of the National University [was] the first panel member and hence the first woman member defeated.'[108]

English's defeat was not, however, the only drama at the National University count:

> As the result of the National University polling was about to be declared in Dublin last night, seven armed men held up the officials and seized all the documents and the result sheets. The officials had taken a copy of the result, which showed the following four candidates elected: – Professors John MacNeil and Hayes, pro-Treaty panel candidates; Professor Stockley, anti-Treaty panel; and Professor Magennis, pro-Treaty independent. The defeated candidates were Dr Ada English, anti-Treaty panel and Professor Conway, pro-Treaty independent. This is a Treaty gain of one.[109]

The *New York Times* reported that the 'sensational raid' was performed by 'Rory O'Connor, the rebel leader of the Four Courts'.[110] O'Connor was an anti-Treaty Republican activist from Dublin. On this occasion, O'Connor's 'thirteen armed men' arrived at the Senate Rooms of the National University 'in two motor cars' just as the count was completed.[111] The leader announced to those present, 'I am sorry, ladies and gentlemen, for disturbing you':

> Seven of them entered the building and held up all the officials and everyone present at the count. They immediately proceeded to seize the voting papers and documents relating to the election, including the results sheets. This clearance was effected very speedily, and after a few minutes they took their departure with the seized documents, the leader stating in a reply to an official, 'We have reason for everything we do'.[112]

The raid prompted precautions at Dublin's other count centres over the following days:

> The ballot boxes containing the votes recorded in yesterday's elections in Dublin City and County have been placed under armed guards of Free State troops in the Drumcondra schools and the Rathmines Town Hall respectively, where the counts will begin at ten o'clock on Monday morning… This precaution is probably consequent upon last night's amazing experience in the Senate Rooms of the National University, when the voting papers were seized by armed men in civilian clothes immediately after the count for that constituency had been completed… The fact that under the special conditions of University polling the papers bore the signatures of the voters is thought to be significant of the purpose of the raid.[113]

Overall, this election was an especially difficult one for O'Connor: some days after the raid at the National University, the *New York Times* reported that the 'defeat of Liam Mellows [at the polls] in Galway' was 'a severe blow to General Rory O'Connor, being the brains of that extreme wing of republicanism'.[114] O'Connor, like Mellows,[115] was executed during the Civil War.

Even with media attention devoted to the drama of the raid, the outcome of the National University count and the defeat of English also provoked comment:

> What is considered to be the most interesting feature of the first issued result of the polls in the Irish elections is the defeat of Dr Ada English,

who was prominent in the Dáil Éireann debates of December and January for her attack on the Treaty.[116]

Constance Markievicz, Kathleen Clarke and Margaret Pearse, who, like English, opposed the Treaty in the Second Dáil, also lost their seats.[117] In Clarke's own words:

> My luck was out in Dublin, I was not re-elected. It did not worry me much; I was in the same boat as the other women TDs who voted against the Treaty, Countess Markievicz, Mrs O'Callaghan, Miss Mary MacSwiney, Dr Ada English and Mrs Pearse. Well, we all paid for our temerity in voting as we did. We were all women who had worked and suffered for the freedom of our country.
>
> The election being over, I had temporarily very little to do. It felt strange having so little to do…[118]

English's seat was taken by Professor William Magennis, an independent candidate. That was to be the last time English ran for elected political office, but it was by no means the end of her political activities: she had much yet to do.

Civil War (1922–3)

In mid-1922, a Civil War broke out between factions that supported and opposed the Treaty. The pro-Treaty side was led by Michael Collins, who became Commander-in-Chief of the National Army in 1922, and Richard Mulcahy, a politician and nationalist who served in the 1916 Easter Rising and was Chief-of-Staff of the IRA during the War of Independence. The anti-Treaty side was led by Liam Lynch, an officer in the IRA during both the War of Independence and Civil War, and Frank Aiken, an IRA commander and, later, holder of multiple ministries in various Irish governments. Predictably, English supported the anti-Treaty side.[119]

The Civil War marked a bitter, divisive period in Irish history. In April 1922 anti-Treaty IRA members occupied the Four Courts in Dublin and a fierce battle ensued. English was in Dublin during this tumultuous period. Mrs Mary Flannery Woods of Rathfarnham, an active member of Cumman na mBan, recalls how she was woken by the 'boom' of the guns bombarding the Four Courts, rushed to Dublin's Quays to liaise with colleagues, and then 'returned to Suffolk Street where I met my husband and Dr English'.[120]

Not all republicans agreed with the occupation of the Four Courts. Cathal Brugha, who had been appointed Chairman of the Resident Executive of the

IRA in 1917, and who opposed the Treaty, also opposed the occupation of the Four Courts. Nonetheless, in order to relieve the relentless pressure on his colleagues there, Brugha and some other anti-Treaty fighters occupied areas around Sackville Street (later O'Connell Street) in Dublin city-centre in June 1922.

It is reported that English served with Brugha at the Hammam Hotel on Sackville Street during this phase of the fighting.[121] English had a close association with Brugha, a man who always acknowledged the key role Irish women played in the struggle for Irish freedom. Following the 1916 Easter Rising, for example, when many of the males leaders were in prison, Brugha appreciated that 'it was the women who kept the spirit alive … kept the flag flying'.[122]

At this point in the Civil War, however, Brugha and his anti-Treaty colleagues were in an extremely difficult position, caught in bitter fighting on Sackville Street. (When the buildings they were in caught fire, many of Brugha's colleagues escaped, including Oscar Traynor, a Dublin-born republican who went on to serve as minister for defence in later years.) Faced with an impossible fight, Brugha ordered his remaining colleagues to surrender but did not do so himself. When Brugha emerged onto the street, he brandished a revolver at Free State troops and was shot in the leg.[123] He was brought to the nearby Mater Misericoridae Hospital where, ironically, English had worked briefly two decades earlier.[124] Despite receiving first aid at the scene of the shooting and undergoing a surgical procedure at the hospital, Brugha died of his injuries on 7 July 1922.[125] His widow specifically requested that members of Cumann na mBan provide the guard of honour at her husband's funeral.[126]

By this time, Irish Free State troops, aided by British artillery, had forced the surrender of anti-Treaty forces occupying the Four Courts and by July 1922 Free State troops had taken general control of Dublin. Anti-Treaty troops dispersed throughout the country and initially held sway in the 'Munster Republic' of Cork, Limerick and Waterford, but were ultimately no match for the Free State troops, who soon took control of all major towns.

Autumn 1922 saw the emergence of more guerrilla warfare tactics in the Civil War, with multiple executions and atrocities perpetrated by both sides. On 22 August 1922 Michael Collins was killed in an ambush at Béal na mBláth in County Cork.[127] In November and December 1922, Free State forces executed several republican leaders, including Liam Mellows, a friend of English and participant in the 1916 Easter Rising in Galway.[128] The anti-Treaty leader, Liam Lynch, was killed in an ambush in County Tipperary on 10 April 1923.[129]

A ceasefire was finally declared on 24 May 1923 and in the subsequent election the pro-Treaty Free State party won 40 per cent of the vote, compared to 27 per cent for the Republicans, represented by Sinn Féin. The Civil War had, however, brought unprecedented division to the country, and left a potent, bitter legacy which was to shape Irish politics for the remainder of the twentieth century and, arguably, beyond.[130]

While it is not entirely clear how many people died as a result of the Civil War, it is likely there were approximately 800 deaths in the Free State army and 400 amongst republicans.[131] In addition, a great many people were taken prisoner, including over 400 republican women, many of whom were members of Cumann na mBan. The British Army file on English records that she, too, was 'arrested by P.G. [Provisional Government; i.e. pro-Treaty] troops, with four other members of Cumann na mBan' in Ballinasloe in August 1922.[132] *Poblacht na hEireann*, the weekly republican newspaper, noted that English 'had also been arrested and imprisoned by the British' in the past.[133] Unlike her experience in 1921 when the British imprisoned her in Galway, there is no record of her being interned by the Free State in 1922.

The Civil War was an especially difficult period for Cumann na mBan, owing not only to divisions about the Treaty within its ranks,[134] but also the fact that many of its members were arrested and then treated poorly while in custody.[135] Margaret Buckley, who was president of Sinn Féin from 1937 to 1950, wrote about conditions of detention for some of these women in Dublin's prisons at the time: 'Máire [Comerford] sat on a bench, like a stoic of old with tightly compressed lips, never emitting even a murmur, while a doctor cut away her hair and put three stitches in her head. I had seen [Sheila] Humphreys being dragged out, half conscious from the blow dealt her when she resisted the search.'[136]

The Civil War, which claimed more lives than the War of Independence, finally ended in May 1923. After this, English, according to her obituary in the *Irish Independent*, 'played no further part in public life'.[137]

Conclusion

Irish nationalist politics clearly played a central part in English's life. She was deeply dedicated to the cause of Irish independence, dating from her earliest contacts with Pearse prior to 1916 and her time with the Irish Volunteers and Cumann na mBan. Her court-martial and imprisonment in Galway jail during the War of Independence were virtually inevitable outcomes of her sustained political activity. English's election to the second Dáil gave her a national platform for her views, and opportunity to support de Valera's nomination as President of the Irish Republic and oppose the Anglo-Irish Treaty. The Civil War saw her return to the republican struggle, at the heart of events in Dublin city centre.

It is not quite true to state, however, that English's political involvements ceased following the end of the Civil War as English remained at least somewhat politically active well into the latter part of the 1920s. On 22 January 1929, for example, the *Irish Times* carried a report titled 'Republicans in the Rotunda: Miss MacSwiney's Dáil in Session':

> Miss Mary MacSwiney and sixteen other members of her political organisation sat in the Pillar Room of the Rotunda, Dublin, yesterday, as the only Simon Pure Dáil Éireann, and solemnly passed the first reading of 'The Constitution of the Republic of Ireland Bill'. A handful of the general public and some uniformed 'Fianna' girl guides formed the audience during the day, but at the night sitting there were about 150 of the general public present… Around the room a member of Cumann na mBan in uniform stood sentry at each pillar… Members of Cumann na mBan also acted as guards and scrutineers at the entrance.[138]

Mary MacSwiney was an Irish politician and educationalist, elected, like English, as a Sinn Féin member of the Second Dáil. She was interned during and after the Civil War, and went on hunger strike. Unlike English, she retained her seat in the Third Dáil for anti-Treaty Sinn Fein, but refused to enter the Dáil, and lost her seat in June 1927. MacSwiney, whose brother Terence died on hunger strike in Brixton Prison during the War of Independence, maintained a hard-line republican stance throughout her life.

In MacSwiney's view, the new Dáil, formed after the Civil War, did not represent a legitimate government for Ireland, and so she established 'Miss MacSwiney's Dáil' as an alternative, *real* government for the country. MacSwiney's 'legislators' included various republicans and anti-Treaty activists who 'adhered to the old Republican programme' and did not recognise the legitimacy of the new Dáil.

In January 1929, MacSwiney's 'legislators' included several familiar names from the history of Irish republicanism, including Kathleen Lynn (see Chapter Four) and Austin Stack, who had offered English promotion to Sligo Mental Hospital in 1921[139] and, like MacSwiney, ceased to be a member of the new Dáil in 1927.

English, consistent with her anti-Treaty stance, was listed as an 'absentee' member of 'Miss MacSwiney's Dáil' in January 1929.[140] Clearly, then, while English was not actually present at the Rotunda meeting, there can be little doubt at which end of the republican spectrum her sympathies still lay. Moreover, in spite of her diminished political activities, English retained some political connections throughout the 1930s: in June 1932, for example, at the start of the Eucharistic Congress of Dublin, English was a guest at a State Reception at Dublin Castle, hosted by her old friend, President de Valera, along with Cardinal Bourne, Archbishop of Westminster and various other religious leaders.[141] Although English had such connections, it remains the case that her active, public political activities diminished substantially following the Civil War.

For Ireland as a country, the Civil War had exerted a huge cost in terms of human, financial and political capital. For English, the Civil War, like the 1916 Easter Rising, had brought yet more personal losses in the cause of Irish nationalism including, most notably, the death of her close associate, Cathal Brugha, in Dublin in July 1922.

For Ireland as a whole, the reconstruction of the country's economy following the Civil War was a deeply challenging task owing not only to the effects of sustained conflict and the recession of the 1930s, but also the development of a trade war with Britain. In 1937 a new constitution was finally passed by referendum but it was not until 1949 that the Republic of Ireland came into being.[142]

Sadly, English did not live to see the establishment of the Irish republic. Throughout her life, however, English had dedicated much of her time and energy to the cause of Irish nationalism, and made a significant contribution to Ireland's search for independence.

From a broader perspective, English's resolutely nationalist outlook not only informed her public political life but also influenced her medical work at Ballinasloe District Asylum, where she combined political activity with progressive medical practice over her four decades at the institution.[143] This dimension of English's life and work is considered next.

Notes

1. *Irish Times*, 5 January 1922.
2. *Irish Press*, 28 January 1944.
3. *Irish Independent*, 27 January 1944.
4. R. Dudley Edwards, *Patrick Pearse: The Triumph of Failure* (Dublin: Irish Academic Press, 2006), p.29.
5. *Irish Times*, 22 November 1934.
6. F. Clarke, 'English, Adeline ('Ada')', in J. McGuire and J. Quinn (eds), *Dictionary of Irish Biography: From the Earliest Times to the Year 2002 (Volume 3, D-F)* (Cambridge: Royal Irish Academy and Cambridge University Press, 2009), pp.626–7.
7. *Irish Press*, 28 January 1944; *East Galway Democrat*, 29 January 1944; McNamara and Mooney, *Women in Parliament: 1918–2000*, p.79.
8. Dudley Edwards, *Patrick Pearse*, p. 29.
9. R. Ellman, *James Joyce (Second Edition)* (Oxford and New York: Oxford University Press, 1984), p. 61.

10. F.O.C. Meenan, *Cecilia Street: The Catholic University School of Medicine, 1855–1931* (Dublin: Gill and Macmillan, 1987), pp.74–5. See also: J.F. Byrne, *Silent Years: An Autobiography with Memoirs of James Joyce and Our Ireland* (New York: Farrar, Strauss and Young, 1953), chapter 12; R. Ellman, *James Joyce (Second Edition)* (Oxford and New York: Oxford University Press, 1984), pp.89, 97, 104–7, 140.
11. Dudley Edwards, *Patrick Pearse*, p. 29.
12. Scoil Éanna Ltd Share Certificate, No. 31, 22 January 1912, PMSTE.2003.864 (Pearse Museum/OPW, St Enda's Park, Grange Road, Rathfarnham, County Dublin, Ireland).
13. McCarthy, *Cumann na mBan and the Irish Revolution*, p.46.
14. Kelly, *Between the Lines of History*, p.25; McNamara and Mooney, *Women in Parliament*, p.79; M. Clancy, 'On the "Western Outpost": Local government and women's suffrage in county Galway', in G. Moran (ed.), *Galway: History and Society – Interdisciplinary Essays on the History of an Irish County* (Dublin: Geography Publications, 1996), pp.557–87; p. 562; Witness Statement (Number 568) of Eilis, Bean Uí Chonaill (Dublin: Bureau of Military History, 1913-21, File Number S.1846), p.55; Witness Statement (Number 1,752) of Mrs McCarvill (Eileen McGrane) (Dublin: Bureau of Military History, 1913-21, File Number S.1434), p.7; *Irish Press*, 28 January 1944; *East Galway Democrat*, 29 January 1944.
15. McCarthy, *Cumann na mBan and the Irish Revolution*, p.9.
16. M.T. Foy and B. Barton, *The Easter Rising* (Dublin: Sutton Publishing, 2004), pp.7–8.
17. Kelly, *Between the Lines of History*, p.25; McNamara and Mooney, *Women in Parliament: 1918–2000*, p.79.
18. McCarthy, *Cumann na mBan and the Irish Revolution*, p.10; *Irish Times*, 26 November 1913.
19. McCarthy, *Cumann na mBan and the Irish Revolution*, p.15.
20. *Irish Times*, 3 April 1914.
21. McCarthy, *Cumann na mBan and the Irish Revolution*, p.10; *Irish Times*, 26 November 1913.
22. McNamara and Mooney, *Women in Parliament*, p.79; Witness Statement (Number 568) of Eilis, Bean Uí Chonaill (Dublin: Bureau of Military History, 1913–21, File Number S.1846), p. 55; Witness Statement (Number 1,752) of Mrs McCarvill (Eileen McGrane) (Dublin: Bureau of Military History, 1913–21, File Number S.1434), p.7; *Irish Press*, 28 January 1944; *East Galway Democrat*, 29 January 1944.
23. T. Mac Loughlin, *Ballinasloe Inniú agus Inné: A Story of a Community Over the Past 300 Years* (Ballinasloe: Tadgh Mac Loughlin, 1993), p.168.
24. McCarthy, *Cumann na mBan and the Irish Revolution*, pp.22–4.
25. A. Matthews, *Renegades: Irish Republican Women, 1900–1922* (Cork: Mercier Press, 2010), p.110; McCarthy, *Cumann na mBan and the Irish Revolution*, p.33.
26. McCarthy, *Cumann na mBan and the Irish Revolution*, p.53.
27. C.D. Greaves, *Liam Mellows and the Irish Revolution* (Belfast: An Ghlór Gafa, 2004).
28. S. McCoole, *No Ordinary Women: Irish Female Activists in the Revolutionary Years, 1900–1923* (Dublin: O'Brien Press, 2003), pp.185–6.
29. Greaves, *Liam Mellows and the Irish Revolution*, p.92.

30. J. Mooney Eichacker, *Irish Republican Women in America: Lecture Tours, 1916–1925* (Dublin: Irish Academic Press, 2003), p.12; McCarthy, *Cumann na mBan and the Irish Revolution*, p.56.

31. L. Conlon, *Cumann na mBan and the Women of Ireland, 1913–1925* (Kilkenny: Kilkenny People Ltd, 1969).

32. Kelly, *Between the Lines of History*, p.25; F. Clarke, 'English, Adeline ('Ada')', in J. McGuire and J. Quinn (eds), *Dictionary of Irish Biography: From the Earliest Times to the Year 2002 (Volume 3, D-F)* (Cambridge: Royal Irish Academy and Cambridge University Press, 2009), pp.626–7.

33. McNamara and Mooney, *Women in Parliament*, p.79; Witness Statement (Number 568) of Eilis, Bean Uí Chonaill (Dublin: Bureau of Military History, 1913–21, File Number S.1846), p.55; Witness Statement (Number 1,752) of Mrs McCarvill (Eileen McGrane) (Dublin: Bureau of Military History, 1913–21, File Number S.1434), p.7; *Irish Press*, 28 January 1944; *East Galway Democrat*, 29 January 1944.

34. *Irish Press*, 28 January 1944.

35. McNamara and Mooney, *Women in Parliament: 1918–2000*, p.79; *Irish Press*, 28 January 1944; *East Galway Democrat*, 29 January 1944.

36. McCarthy, *Cumann na mBan and the Irish Revolution*, pp.63–4.

37. S. O'Dubhghaill, 'Activities in Enniscorthy', *The Capuchin Annual*, 1966.

38. *Irish Times*, 29 January 1944.

39. *East Galway Democrat*, 29 January 1944.

40. Witness Statement (Number 806) of Mrs George Clancy (Máire, Bean Mhic Fhlannachadha) (Dublin: Bureau of Military History, 1913–21, File Number S.2117), pp.3, 15.

41. Greaves, *Liam Mellows and the Irish Revolution*, p.390.

42. McCarthy, *Cumann na mBan and the Irish Revolution*, p.72.

43. McCoole, *No Ordinary Women*, pp.51–58.

44. Ibid., pp.185–6.

45. War Office, 'Castle File No. 4168: Dr English, Ada', WO 35/206/75 (Kew Richmond, Surrey: British National Archives), p.1.

46. M. Mac Curtain, *Ariadne's Thread: Writing Women into Irish History* (Galway: Arlen House, 2008), p.95.

47. Coogan, *De Valera*.

48. *East Galway Democrat*, 29 January 1944.

49. McNamara and Mooney, *Women in Parliament: 1918–2000*, p.79.

50. *Irish Press*, 28 January 1944; McNamara and Mooney, *Women in Parliament: 1918–2000*, p.79; F. Clarke, 'English, Adeline ('Ada')', in J. McGuire and J. Quinn (eds), *Dictionary of Irish Biography*, pp.626–7.

51. *East Galway Democrat*, 29 January 1944; *Irish Press*, 28 January 1944; McNamara and Mooney, *Women in Parliament: 1918–2000*, p.79.

52. Kelly, *Between the Lines of History*, p.25.

53. McCarthy, *Cumann na mBan and the Irish Revolution*, pp.125–33.

54. Witness Statement (Number 1,752) of Mrs McCarvill (Eileen McGrane) (Dublin: Bureau of Military History, 1913-21, File Number S.1434), p.7; *Irish Press*, 28 January 1944.

55. War Office, 'Castle File No. 4168: Dr English, Ada', p.1.

56. M. Hopkinson, *The Irish War of Independence* (Dublin: Gill and Macmillan Limited, 2004), pp.201–2.

57. Witness Statement (Number 1,062) of Laurence Garvey (Dublin: Bureau of Military History, 1913-21, File Number S.2367), pp. 11-12.

58. *Irish Times*, 20 January 1921.

59. *Western News and Galway Leader*, 22 January 1921.

60. P. Lavelle, *James O'Mara: The Story of an Original Sinn Féiner* (Ireland: The History Publisher, 2011); p.207.

61. Witness Statement (Number 366) of Alice M. Cashel (Dublin: Bureau of Military History, 1913–21, File Number S.1420), p.9.

62. Ibid.

63. McNamara and Mooney, *Women in Parliament: 1918–2000*, p.79; *Irish Press*, 28 January 1944; *East Galway Democrat*, 29 January 1944.

64. Greaves, *Liam Mellows and the Irish Revolution*, p.390.

65. General Register of Prisoners, Galway Prison, 1921 (National Archives, Bishop Street, Dublin, Ireland).

66. Witness Statement (Number 366) of Alice M. Cashel (Dublin: Bureau of Military History, 1913–21, File Number S.1420), p.10.

67. Lavelle, *James O'Mara: The Story of an Original Sinn Féiner*, pp.207–8.

68. General Register of Prisoners, Galway Prison, 1921 (National Archives, Bishop Street, Dublin, Ireland); *Irish Times*, 25 February 1921.

69. General Register of Prisoners, Galway Prison, 1921 (National Archives, Bishop Street, Dublin, Ireland); War Office, 'Castle File No. 4168: Dr English, Ada', p.1.

70. *Irish Times*, 12 March 1921.

71. General Register of Prisoners, Galway Prison, 1921 (National Archives, Bishop Street, Dublin, Ireland).

72. Witness Statement (Number 366) of Alice M. Cashel (Dublin: Bureau of Military History, 1913–21, File Number S.1420), p.10.

73. *Western News and Galway Leader*, 26 February 1921.

74. Matthews, *Renegades*, p.262.

75. McCoole, *No Ordinary Women*, p.80.

76. *Irish Press*, 28 January 1944.

77. G. Plunkett Dillon (edited by H. O Brolchain), *All in the Blood: A Memoir of the Plunkett Family, the 1916 Rising and the War of Independence* (Dublin: A. & A. Farmar, 2006), p.304.

78. General Register of Prisoners, Galway Prison, 1921 (National Archives, Bishop Street, Dublin, Ireland).

79. *East Galway Democrat*, 29 January 1944; War Office, 'Castle File No. 4168: Dr English, Ada', p.1.

80. *Western News and Galway Leader,* 11 June 1921.

81. War Office, 'Castle File No. 4168: Dr English, Ada', p.1.

82. M. Clancy, 'Shaping the Nation: Women in the Free State Parliament', in Y. Galligan, E. Ward and R. Wilford (eds), *Contesting Politics: Women in Ireland, North and South* (Boulder, Colorado: Westview Press, 1999), pp.201–18; p.205.

83. A. Griffith, *The Resurrection of Hungary: A Parallel for Ireland* (Dublin: Patrick Mahon, 1904), p.161.

84. *Irish Press*, 28 January 1944.
85. Witness Statement (Number 1,219) of Sean O'Neill (Dublin: Bureau of Military History, 1913–21, File Number S.2451), p.46.
86. Mac Loughlin, *Ballinasloe Inniú agus Inné*, p.168; F. Clarke, 'English, Adeline ('Ada')', in J. McGuire and J. Quinn (eds), *Dictionary of Irish Biography*, pp.626–7.
87. Witness Statement (Number 568) of Eilis, Bean Uí Chonaill (Dublin: Bureau of Military History, 1913–21, File Number S.1846), p. 55. See also: *Irish Times*, 29 January 1944.
88. *The Times*, 16 May 1921.
89. *Official Report of Dáil Éireann*, 4 January 1922.
90. J. Knirk, *Women of the Dáil: Gender, Republicanism and the Anglo-Irish Treaty* (Dublin: Irish Academic Press, 2006), pp.16–17; M. Ward, 'Times of transition: Republican women, feminism and political representation', in L. Ryan and M. Ward (eds), *Irish Women and Nationalism: Soldiers, New Women and Wicked Hags* (Dublin: Irish Academic Press, 2004), pp.184–201; p.189.
91. War Office, 'Castle File No. 4168: Dr English, Ada', p.1.
92. *Official Report of Dáil Éireann*, 26 August 1921.
93. *Irish Times*, 29 January 1944.
94. T.P. Coogan, *Michael Collins: A Biography* (London: Arrow Books, 1991).
95. *Gloucester Citizen,* 21 September 1921. For further reports on this meeting, see: *Derby Daily Telegraph*, 21 September 1921; *Evening Telegraph – Dundee*, 21 September 1921; *Hull Daily Mail*, 21 September 1921; Nottingham *Evening Post*, 21 September 1921; *Western Times – Exeter*, 22 September 1921.
96. *Official Report of Dáil Éireann*, 4 January 1922.
97. Eichacker, *Irish Republican Women in America*, p.21; Ward, *Irish Women and Nationalism*; p.190.
98. Knirk, *Women of the Dáil*, pp.85, 100.
99. McCoole, *No Ordinary Women*, p.86; G. Kearns, 'Mother Ireland and the revolutionary sisters', *Cultural Geographies*, 11, 4 (October 2004), pp.443–67.
100. *Official Report of Dáil Éireann*, 4 January 1922.
101. *Irish Times*, 5 January 1922. See also: *Aberdeen Daily Journal*, 5 January 1922.
102. *Irish Times*, 5 January 1922.
103. *Irish Times*, 9 January 1922.
104. Ferriter, *The Transformation of Ireland 1900–2000*, p.247.
105. *Irish Times*, 10 June 1922.
106. *Irish Times*, 19 June 1922 & 24 June 1922.
107. *Aberdeen Daily Journal*, 17 June 1922.
108. *New York Times*, 18 June 1922; *Irish Times*, 17 June 1922.
109. *Western Daily Press – Bristol*, 17 June 1922.
110. *New York Times*, 17 June 1922.
111. *Aberdeen Daily Journal,* 17 June 1922.
112. Ibid.
113. *Sunday Post – Glasgow*, 18 June 1922. See also: *Western Daily Press – Bristol,* 19 June 1922.
114. *New York Times*, 21 June 1922.
115. Greaves, *Liam Mellows and the Irish Revolution*, p.390.

116. *Sunday Post – Glasgow*, 18 June 1922. See also: *Western Daily Press – Bristol*, 19 June 1922.
117. McCoole, *No Ordinary Women*, p.90; F. Clarke, 'English, Adeline ('Ada')', in J. McGuire and J. Quinn (eds), *Dictionary of Irish Biography*, pp. 626–7.
118. K. Clarke (edited by H. Litton), *Revolutionary Woman: My Fight for Ireland's Freedom* (Dublin: The O'Brien Press, 1991), p.196
119. *Irish Press*, 28 January 1944; McNamara and Mooney, *Women in Parliament: 1918–2000*, p.79.
120. Witness Statement (Number 624) of Mrs Mary Flannery Woods (Dublin: Bureau of Military History, 1913–21, File Number S.1901), pp.66–8.
121. *Irish Press*, 28 January 1944; McNamara and Mooney, *Women in Parliament: 1918–2000*, p.79; F. Clarke, 'English, Adeline ('Ada')', in J. McGuire and J. Quinn (eds), *Dictionary of Irish Biography*, pp.626–7.
122. M. Ward, *Unmanageable Revolutionaries: Women in Irish Nationalism* (London: Pluto Press, 1995), p.123.
123. *Irish Times*, 2 September 2008.
124. *Irish Times*, 29 January 1944.
125. *Irish Times*, 18 August 2008; *Irish Times*, 2 September 2008.
126. McCarthy, *Cumann na mBan and the Irish Revolution*, pp.200–1.
127. Coogan, *Michael Collins*.
128. *Irish Times*, 29 January 1944.
129. Ferriter, *The Transformation of Ireland 1900–2000*, p. 265.
130. Ibid., pp.268–9.
131. Ibid., p.258.
132. War Office, 'Castle File No. 4168: Dr English, Ada', p.1.
133. *Poblacht na hEireann: War News*, 10 August 1922.
134. McCarthy, *Cumann na mBan and the Irish Revolution*, pp.194–8.
135. A. Matthews, *Dissidents: Irish Republican Women, 1923–1941* (Cork: Mercier Press, 2012), pp.44–119.
136. M. Buckley, *The Jangle of the Keys* (Dublin: Duffy and Company, 1938), p.50; Ferriter, *The Transformation of Ireland 1900–2000*, p.269.
137. *Irish Independent*, 27 January 1944.
138. *Irish Times*, 22 January 1929.
139. *East Galway Democrat*, 29 January 1944; McNamara and Mooney, *Women in Parliament: 1918–2000*, p.79.
140. *Irish Times*, 22 January 1929.
141. *Irish Times*, 22 June 1932.
142. Ferriter, *The Transformation of Ireland 1900–2000*, p.258.
143. *Irish Times*, 29 January 1944.

CHAPTER THREE

———— ❧ ☙ ————

Medicine: Psychiatry and the Asylum, 1904–42

Thanks to the indifference of the public, our asylums are in a bad way. They are over-crowded. They are both understaffed and inefficiently staffed. Curable and incurable cases are herded together. There is practically no treatment. The percentage of cures remains at a very low figure. Public money is wasted. The asylums are unsuited for their purpose in almost every respect.

Edward Boyd Barrett (1924)[1]

In 1904, English went to work at Ballinasloe District Asylum, later renamed St Brigid's Hospital (1960), in Ballinasloe, County Galway. Forty years later, English's obituary in the *East Galway Democrat* stated that she 'gave her life's professional work to Ballinasloe and Castlerea Mental Hospitals', becoming Resident Medical Superintendent at Ballinasloe in 1941, just three years prior to her death.[2]

The *Irish Press* wrote that English 'was foremost in urging and helping the changes which transformed the then "Lunatic Asylum" to be one of the finest mental hospitals in the country. She developed occupational therapy to a high degree, and Ballinasloe was the first mental hospital in Ireland to start electric convulsive therapy.'[3] Today, English is still remembered as both a nationalist politician and a pioneering doctor.[4]

English's decision to devote her medical skills to working in asylums was an interesting one. The entry of women into medicine during this period was, for the most part, associated with other areas of medical practice, such as infant healthcare and public health.[5] Dr Kathleen Lynn, for example, graduated from the Royal University in 1899 and co-founded St Ultan's Hospital for Infants in 1919, resulting in substantial improvements in infant and child health in Dublin.[6] Dr Dorothy Price, another pioneering female doctor, graduated from the University of Dublin (Trinity College) in 1921 and played a key role in the eradication of tuberculosis in Ireland, resulting in substantial public health benefit.[7] Interestingly, both of these doctors were, like English, highly politically active (see Chapter Four).

It is possible that English was attracted to asylums because of clear evidence of unmet need amongst the mentally ill, compounded by inexorable growth in asylum populations throughout the nineteenth and early twentieth centuries.[8] This chapter examines these trends as a background to English's arrival in Ballinasloe in 1904, and explores her work in the asylum up until her retirement in 1942. This was a time of great activity both at the asylum in Ballinasloe and throughout Irish mental health services in general. English made many contributions to both.

Mental Health Services in Early Twentieth-Century Ireland

The decades preceding the start of English's career in the asylums in 1904 saw substantial change in Irish mental health services. In the early part of the nineteenth century, there had been scant provision for individuals with mental illness in Ireland, many of whom were either homeless, residing in workhouses, or admitted to the small number of public and private asylums that existed at that time.[9]

Notwithstanding the opening of Cork Lunatic Asylum in 1791[10] and the Richmond Asylum, Dublin in 1814,[11] it was apparent that systematic reform at national level was needed. As a result, a bill to establish a system of asylums was presented to parliament by William Vesey Fitzgerald, a British politician and administrator, and passed on 11 July 1817.[12] The remainder of the nineteenth century was a time of intensive legislative and building activity, resulting in the establishment of a substantial network of asylums across Ireland,[13] analogous to that in England.[14]

In 1825, the first of the new wave of asylums was established in Armagh and this was followed by asylums in Clonmel, Limerick, Ballinasloe, Waterford, Belfast, Carlow, Derry, Maryborough, Kilkenny, Letterkenny, Killarney, Cork, Mullingar, Castlebar, Sligo, Omagh, Ennis, Downpatrick, Monaghan and Enniscorthy.[15] The intense building programme resulted in a large increase in the number of public asylum beds: in 1830 there were just 791 asylum beds for 'pauper lunatics' in Ireland and by 1896 this had risen to 13,620.[16]

In 1838, the Criminal Lunatics (Ireland) Act was passed, permitting the transfer of an individual to an asylum if they were considered dangerous and either mentally ill or intellectually disabled. This soon became the admission pathway of choice, chiefly because it dispensed with the need for a certificate of poverty and gave police full responsibility for transporting the individual to the asylum, which was then under an obligation to admit the individual.[17] As a result, the 'dangerous lunacy' procedure was widely abused and contributed significantly to the rise in committals as the 1800s progressed.[18]

In the midst of this activity, the Connaught District Lunatic Asylum was opened in Ballinasloe in 1833 at a cost of £27,000.[19] The governors and directors were appointed by the Lord Lieutenant of Ireland and included prominent churchmen, titled land-owners and Members of Parliament. Both a medical officer and manager were appointed from the start.

The asylum in Ballinasloe had capacity for 150 patients and initially catered for Galway, Roscommon, Sligo, Leitrim and Mayo. In 1855, an asylum was completed in Sligo (to cater for Sligo and Leitrim) and in 1861 an asylum opened in Castlebar (to cater for Mayo). As a result, Connaught District Lunatic Asylum was renamed Ballinasloe District Asylum and catered only for patients from Galway and Roscommon.

As with many district asylums, the institution in Ballinasloe experienced strong demand for beds and a new wing was added to the male side in 1871, followed by an extension to the female side in 1882.[20] A Roman Catholic chapel was also added. However, the resident medical superintendent (RMS), Dr Fletcher,[21] reported to the Ballinasloe Board of Governors in 1885 that there still was a significant problem with overcrowding:

> Whatever was the reason, lunacy was increasing in the district, and Ballinasloe which was originally intended to hold all the lunatics in the province was found inadequate for those of two counties. Even if the governors ordered the erection of the new wing that day it would not be ready for the reception of patients for two years, and provision should be made in the meantime for the accommodation of those over and above the requirements of the institution. Owing to the overcrowded state of the house typhoid fever had broken out, and there had been already thirteen cases. There was another case of fever at present in the house, which he attributed to no other reason than that of overcrowding.[22]

By the 1880s the number of patients had risen to 527, necessitating further additions to the buildings in 1884 and 1888. By 1892 the number of patients had risen yet again to 791 (472 male, 319 female).[23] In that year, the Inspectors of Lunatics reported significant problems with overcrowding throughout all of Ireland's district asylum network:

> The accommodation in District Asylums in this country still continues quite inadequate to supply the wants of the insane population. We have again to repeat the statement made in former reports that the overcrowding is rapidly increasing, and that the necessity for further accommodation is becoming more and more urgent.[24]

By 1896, there were 935 patients in Ballinasloe, and there were plans for yet another extension. The new block, detached from the main hospital, was opened in 1901 and the number of patients reached 1,004.[25]

The intense pressure on asylum beds during this period was most likely related to a combination of factors including changing diagnostic practices, philanthropic impulses, legislative change, socio-economic difficulties and possible changes in the epidemiology of illnesses such as schizophrenia.[26] The absence of effective treatments undoubtedly also contributed to the problem. The process of industrialisation, too, tended to diminish the capacity of families to care for individuals with mental illness resulting in greater pressure on asylum beds. Similarly, emigration, especially in the 1840s and 1850s, eroded families' abilities to manage individuals with mental illness or intellectual disability in their homes or on their farms, further increasing pressure on the asylums.

Whatever the reasons for this trend, it was clear there was a serious problem with overcrowding in Irish asylums, including Ballinasloe.[27] In 1903, the year before English commenced working in Ballinasloe and the year in which she served as a clinical assistant at the vast Richmond Asylum in Dublin,[28] a Conference of the Irish Asylums Committee was convened at the Richmond to consider the inexorable rise in demand for asylum beds.[29] There were, however, no ready solutions to the growing crisis and, by 1914, there were 16,941 individuals resident in Irish district asylums; this figure was to continue to rise until the late 1950s, interrupted only by two short-lived declines during the two World Wars. It was this system of custodial psychiatry, with its vast and expanding institutions, into which English entered in 1904.

Politics in the Asylum

In September 1904, when English sought work in Ballinasloe District Asylum, there were 1,293 patients there (774 male, 519 female) and, of these, 311 were described as being 'under treatment' (203 male, 108 female).[30] In June 1904,

English had applied, unsuccessfully, for 'the post of second assistant medical officer' in Ballinasloe,[31] but she applied again later that year and her second application was considered with great care by the Committee of Management on 12 September 1904.

The minutes of this meeting record that 'applications for the post of second assistant medical officer in this asylum from Doctors Ada English, G.W. Downing and Malone Lee having been read, the Most Rev F.J. McCormack DD proposed … the appointment of Dr Ada English…'[32] The Committee of Management voted on the matter and English was the clear winner, with eighteen votes, as compared to three for Dr Malone Lee.

Earlier in 1904, there had been considerable controversy over the appointment of a new RMS in Ballinasloe.[33] The two doctors involved were Dr Mills, a Protestant who had been employed in the asylum since May 1893[34] and had been acting RMS for four months, and Dr Richard Kirwan, a Roman Catholic who was 'junior assistant' to Mills.[35] Kirwan was proposed for the post by the Bishop of Galway, who 'presided over the Asylum Committee'. The 'seconder of the Bishop's proposition to appoint Kirwan gave as a reason for that motion that ninety-six per cent of the inmates were Roman Catholics, and the medical superintendent ought, therefore, to be Catholic also'.

Predictably, this appointment caused considerable controversy. The matter was raised in the House of Commons in July 1904 where it was noted that 'Dr Mills was possessed of all the qualifications necessary' but appeared to have been passed over on religious grounds.[36] It transpired that the Lord Lieutenant (chief administrator of British government in Ireland) had already 'sent to ask the reasons of the appointment, and the [Ballinasloe Asylum] Committee came to the conclusion that the Lord Lieutenant had no right to ask them for any reason'. Nonetheless, the Lord Lieutenant 'wanted the Chief Secretary to tell them whether the action of the Asylum Committee was the result of religious feeling, and was it taken because Dr Mills was a Protestant'.

During the heated debate, the House of Commons heard vivid evidence of Kirwan's political leanings:

> The first thing Dr Kirwan did after his appointment to prove his suitability was to take out the emblem of England from the standard of the asylum. He admitted that he did it, and when the attendants of the asylum were receiving their uniforms he was so faithful to his creed that the buttons had to have the harp and shamrock only upon them.[37]

The House of Commons was reassured that 'by law the Ballinasloe Asylum was allowed to choose its own superintendent. They chose Kirwan, and the Lord

Lieutenant felt, after investigation and inquiry, there was not a sufficiently strong case to over-rule the committee.' The debate was nonetheless very heated and, in the words of one participant, 'one would have imagined that they were not in the House of Commons, but were in Ballinasloe Lunatic Asylum – *(Oh, oh, and laughter)* – because he had never in his experience of the House of Commons witnessed a more grotesque exhibition than that to which the House had just listened.'

Later that year, English was appointed to work in Ballinasloe and, from her earliest days, her political interests were clearly consistent with those of Kirwan.[38] Like Kirwan, English supported the move to have the Galway Arms emblazoned in place of Queen Victoria on the buttons of the uniforms in Ballinasloe[39] and promoted the use of Irish-manufactured products in the institution.[40] Like English, Kirwan was deeply involved in a broad range of nationalist activities, and strongly associated the Ballinasloe branch of Conradh na Gaeilge (Gaelic League), an Irish language organisation founded in 1893 by Dubhghlas de hÍde (Douglas Hyde), who would later become the first president of Ireland (1938–45).

In her early years in Ballinasloe, English befriended various powerful local figures in the nationalist movement, including Dr John Dignan, later Bishop of the Diocese of Clonfert (1924–53).[41] Dignan was a native of Ballygar, County Galway and president of St Joseph's College, The Pines, Ballinasloe from 1904 to 1919.[42] Both Dignan and English were prominent in the establishment of Sinn Féin in Ballinasloe in 1910[43] and, like Kirwan, both were active in the Gaelic League.[44]

Dignan was elected president of the East Galway branch of Sinn Féin in 1917 and played an important role in establishing Sinn Féin Courts in County Galway. Like English, Dignan had his house raided in 1921, although Dignan was apparently tipped off by the RIC ahead of time. The influence of English, along with that of Fr Patrick Connolly, a priest of the diocese, played a key role in Bishop Dignan's increasingly nationalistic outlook throughout the 1920s.[45]

Throughout this period, English was also a close friend of several leading political figures at national level, including Joseph McDonagh, Patrick Pearse and Arthur Griffith. She is reported to have provided asylum to Liam Mellows and Éamon de Valera in Ballinasloe on several occasions.[46] In addition, a branch of Cumann na mBan was set up in the asylum with English as chairperson.[47]

Happily for English, her nationalist political views were in close accord with those of the Committee of Management, which was strongly nationalist in outlook. Minutes from its meeting of 12 June 1916, for example, record that the following resolution was passed by the Committee:

> That we the members of the Committee of Management of the Ballinasloe
> Asylum, representing both the counties of Galway and Roscommon,
> determinedly protest against the exclusion of any portion of Ulster from
> the scheme of national government now about to be established in this
> country, and we call upon Mr John Redmond and the Irish party to
> oppose anything that would bring about an accentuation of the religious
> bitterness that apparently exists between the north and the rest of Ireland.
> We are willing to concede anything in justice to the bona-fide fears of
> our northern fellow countrymen, but the division of Ireland we will not
> have.[48]

The Committee agreed that copies of this resolution would 'be sent to Prime
Minister, Mr David Lloyd George, and Mr John Redmond', a moderate Irish
nationalist politician. This strongly nationalist tone persisted into the 1920s:
at its meeting on 11 July 1921, the Committee resolved that 'henceforth no
communication of any kind be forwarded to any department of the British
Government in Ireland'.[49]

After English was arrested in 1921, the minutes of the Committee merely
record that Mills, who had become RMS in 1916,[50] informed them that 'Dr
English is under detention in a government institution, consequently I engaged
the services of Dr Ward as locum tenens'.[51] Following her release, English
resumed her duties at the hospital with no apparent difficulties.

The Ballinasloe asylum committee was by no means unique in its nationalist
stance and tone. Management committees appointed in Carlow and various
other asylums after 1898 tended to be of similar mind, consistent with the
generally democratized and nationalist nature of Irish local government at this
time.[52] As a result of these local and national factors, the political atmosphere
in the Ballinasloe asylum was strongly consistent with English's political views
and activities.

Caring for the Mentally Ill

The establishment of the Irish asylums in the 1800s was accompanied by a
clear commitment to the 'moral management' paradigm of treatment.[53] This
approach was predicated on the idea that 'insanity' found its roots in disorders
of the emotions and thoughts, and that traditional medical treatment and
physical restraints may not be appropriate. Its principles included the idea that
the doctor should speak with the patient in a rational fashion, and the patient
should have a healthy diet, exercise frequently and, where possible, engage in a
gainful occupation.

In Cork, Dr William Saunders Hallaran was an early exponent of this approach in Ireland.[54] Hallaran wrote of his methods in his 1810 text book, titled *An Inquiry into the Causes producing the Extraordinary Addition to the Number of Insane together with Extended Observations on the Cure of Insanity with hints as to the Better Management of Public Asylums for Insane Persons*:

> Maniacs, when in a state to be influenced by moral agents, are not to be *subdued ex efficio*, by measures of mere force, and he who will attempt to impose upon their credulity by aiming it at too great a refinement in address or intellect, will often find himself detected, and treated by them with marked contempt… I have in consequence made it a special point on my *review days*, to converse for a few minutes with each patient, on the subject which appeared to be most welcome to his humour. By a regular attention to the duties of this *parade*, I am generally received with as much politeness and decorum as if every individual attached to it had a share of expectancy from the manner in which he may happen to acquit himself on the occasion. The mental exertion employed amongst the convalescents by this species of address is very remarkable, and the advantages flowing from it are almost incredible.[55]

Hallaran also discussed 'removing the convalescent, and incurable insane, to convenient distances from large cities and towns, to well enclosed farms, properly adapted to the purposes of employing them with effect, in the different branches of husbandry and horticulture'. Patients in the asylum 'might on convalescence, be conveyed in covered carriages to the farms, each of which, holding an intimate communication with, and depending on the original foundation, should make daily returns of their proceedings to the principal master, for the weekly inspection of the board of trustees, according to the present invariable custom in this city'.[56]

Jean-Étienne Dominique Esquirol, a French psychiatrist, described moral treatment as 'the application of the faculty of intelligence and of emotions in the treatment of mental alienation'.[57] Today, such an approach would likely be described as '*milieu* therapy' involving the establishment of therapeutic communities and a group-based approach to recovery.[58] As the 1800s progressed, however, the relatively enlightened principles of moral management became less apparent[59] so that the asylum into which English entered in Ballinasloe in 1904 bore little resemblance to the idealised moral management institutions of the 1800s.

There were many reasons for the decline of moral management. In the first instance, Ireland's asylums continually grew in size and were soon overcrowded, with the result that attention was diverted away from the relatively enlightened moral management approach and towards the management of the increasingly large institutions themselves. Key institutional issues included the regulation of large numbers of patients within enclosed spaces, the spread of infectious diseases within asylum buildings, and the ever-increasing pressure on beds. In addition, a renewed emphasis on biological treatments soon emerged, especially at the start of the 1900s, leading to the relative decline of moral management.[60]

The spirit of moral management was not, however, completely extinguished. Throughout the first half of the 1900s, many of its key ideas, especially its focus on exercise and gainful occupation, simply re-emerged in a new form in many asylums, including Ballinasloe, under the new title 'occupational therapy'. In Ireland, the institution leading the way in this field was Killarney Mental Hospital where, in 1933, Dr Eamonn O'Sullivan established an occupational therapy department, following his visits to several European hospitals that already had programmes of occupational therapy in place.[61] O'Sullivan also went on to write an influential textbook on the subject, titled *Textbook of Occupational Therapy: With Chief Reference to Psychological Medicine*.[62]

In Ballinasloe, occupational therapy was actively developed during English's four decades there, especially throughout the 1920s and 1930s. This was one of English's key contributions to the asylum: following her death in 1944, the *East Galway Democrat* recorded that English 'was foremost in urging and helping the changes which transformed the then "lunatic asylum" into one of the finest in the country. She developed occupational therapy to a high degree'.[63]

English was especially concerned that asylum patients should be gainfully occupied and, as a result, their activities on the asylum farms included 'sowing potatoes, mangolds and turnips. They were also employed making fences...'[64] The asylum farm at Ballinasloe was the subject of particular attention in July 1917 when the Summer Meeting of the Irish Division of the Medico-Psychological Association of Great Britain and Ireland was held in Ballinasloe 'by the kind invitation of Dr John Mills (Medical Superintendent)'.

The *Journal of Mental Science* recorded the events of the day in some detail:

> On arrival of the early train from Dublin, Dr Mills met attending members and motored them to the Asylum. After inspecting the farms and wards of the Asylum, the visitors were driven to see various places of interest in the neighbourhood, including the battlefield of Aughrim, returning to the Asylum for luncheon.[65]

There were only five attendees at the meeting: Mills, English, Dr Greene (from Carlow), Dr Gavin (Mullingar) and Dr Richard Leeper (honorary secretary).

Leeper would later go on to become president of the Medico-Psychological Association in 1931.[66] 'Owing to the small attendance,' at the 1917 meeting, 'it was decided that the reading of a paper by Dr Mills on an interesting subject which was on the agenda should be postponed until the Autumn Meeting.' Toward the end of the meeting, Greene drew particular attention to the asylum farm at Ballinasloe:

> Dr I. Adrian Greene, in a short speech, expressed the regret of those present that so few of the members had been able to attend the meeting owing to war conditions, and cordially thanked Dr Mills for his hospitality. He said they had all seen that day the many improvements recently made in the Asylum, and especially the increased food production by the cultivation of the extensive farms they had visited. Dr Gavin having also spoken, and thanked Dr Mills for his kindness and hospitality and for the pleasant and instructive day he had given to his visitors, the proceedings terminated.[67]

The emphasis on gainful activity for patients persisted throughout the 1920s and 1930s. In 1937, for example, female patients were engaged in making rugs, flowers, cardigans, and tapestry, and sewing and crochet work. In addition to working on the farm, the men played football and tennis, and there were billiard tables, cards and musical instruments for amusement. Despite the inevitable overcrowding, 'the medical officers and staff are very kind and devoted to the patients and [the Inspector] was much impressed at the confidence shown by the patients in the staff'.[68]

In 1939, the Inspector made particular reference to the 'occupational therapy department of the hospital' in Ballinasloe, noting that 'a total of 996 patients are engaged in various occupations, as many as 250 being employed on the farm; others are engaged at various trades and handicrafts... The amusements – both indoor and outdoor – of the patients are well catered for; dances are held weekly during the winter months'.[69]

In addition, English was interested in providing appropriate living facilities for the patients, objecting, for example, to inadequate bedding.[70] English was also keen that patients would have sufficient activities and amusements. She was deeply involved in the hospital drama group, along with Kirwan.[71] English also advocated tirelessly that patients should have opportunity to go to the cinema both within the asylum and in Ballinasloe town. In 1940, shortly after her appointment as acting RMS, English requested 'permission for the patients to be allowed out to the cinema in town as our own is not working'.[72] By the following month, she reported to the Committee of Management that 'about 200 patients attend the cinema each Sunday afternoon in the town'.[73]

In October 1940, she pointed out to the Committee that 'it would be a great boon to the patients if the old cinema could be adjusted to take *talkies* [films with sound]'.[74]

English was a strong promoter of sports in the asylum. In 1915 she was largely responsible for the introduction of camogie and the hospital team duly became one of the best in the country.[75] In 1921 a cinder track was laid for the purpose of cycling competitions and National Cycling Championships were later held there. These innovations were strongly consistent with the importance many asylums attached to sport as both an important activity for patients and staff, and a form of therapy.[76] In Ballinasloe, sport had, for many decades, served as an important way for patients to engage with each other and staff, and even create a bridge to the world outside the asylum walls.[77]

The asylum in Ballinasloe had an especially strong tradition of Gaelic games during English's time there. This tradition even influenced recruitment practices: in 1911, Kirwan, who was then RMS in Ballinasloe, recruited Mr John Hanniffy and Mr Bill Fallon, both well-known hurlers with Kilconieron Gaelic Athletic Association (GAA) club near Loughrea, to training–nursing posts at the asylum.[78] The GAA Club was not at all pleased to lose two of its best players, but it was all part of the build–up of nationalist sentiment in Ballinasloe, carefully orchestrated by Kirwan and English. Hanniffy went on to become assistant land steward and spent much time as acting land steward, owing to the prolonged and frequent absences of the land steward, Mr Thomas Murray.

Gaelic games assumed huge importance in the asylum during this period: on 13 June 1914 the *East Galway Democrat* reported 'great excitement over coming match between Asylum and Cullagh', the 'last battle in the St Grellan League':

> The last chime of the three o'clock on Sunday will signal thirty stalwart Gaels to battle. Sixty minutes of excitement! Only a mite of Time to decide whether bonfires will blaze on the plains of Cullagh or the Asylum buildings quake with the powerful vibrations of victory's cheer! One brief hour will solve the problem – 'Who'll win the Cup?'[79]

In most asylums, both staff and patients participated in sports, and sport sometimes acted as an important leveller of relations between staff and patients.[80] In the early 1900s, the asylum in Ballinasloe had especially strong teams in camogie, hockey and tug-of-war, all of which competed nationally.[81] In a moment that undoubtedly pleased English, the asylum tug-of-war team even defeated RIC men in a particularly intense competition.

English herself also participated in sports. She played golf at Ballinasloe Golf Club and, in 1907, the *Irish Times* records that 'Dr Ada English (3) beat Miss Connaughton (6) by 3 and 2.'[82] Later that day, in the Ladies' Semi-Final, English 'beat Miss Leonard (3 up)' but, sadly, the final saw 'Miss K Newell beat Dr English, on the 20th green.'

Medical Treatments at the Asylum

In 1916, when she was still second assistant medical officer, English applied for promotion to the post of RMS at Ballinasloe. At an extraordinary meeting of the Committee of Management, however, Dr John Mills, acting RMS, was proposed for the post, and 'Dr Richard Kirwan and Dr English, the other candidates present, requested to be allowed to withdraw their applications in favour of Dr Mills'.[83] The proceedings and outcome of the meeting were vividly recounted in the *Irish Times*:

> The applications for the vacant position were those of Dr John Mills, who had been for twenty-three years assistant medical officer; Dr Ada English, second assistant medical officer; and an army medical officer at present serving at the front. Drs Kirwan and English stated that they wished to withdraw, and the chairman declared, amidst loud applause, that Dr Mills was unanimously elected.
>
> An extraordinary scene ensued. The news quickly reached the inmates of the institution and loud cheers could be heard from all parts of the building. Several of the patients came from the dining hall and demanded the doctor's presence. On emerging from the boardroom he was seized by the patients who put him on their shoulders, and amidst great cheering he was carried through the corridors.
>
> Dr Ada English was unanimously elected assistant medical officer at a salary of £280 per year with allowances and it was agreed to advertise for a third medical assistant at a salary of £150, with £100 for allowances.[84]

In 1921, English declined a senior position at Sligo Mental Hospital, preferring instead to stay with her patients in Ballinasloe.[85] As a result, English continued to work at Ballinasloe District Asylum throughout the 1920s, 1930s and early 1940s.

In addition to the development of occupational therapy and provision of appropriate leisure activities for patients, Ballinasloe District Asylum was also to the forefront of introducing novel medical treatments for mental illness throughout the early decades of the twentieth century. In 1939, for example,

Dr Bernard Lyons, who became RMS in 1937, reported to the Committee of Management that:

> Dr James Clyne, who acted as locum here before, and who is after having six months special training in modern treatments of mental patients in Cardiff Mental Hospital, is acting as locum. I am availing of this opportunity of trying some of the new treatments in this hospital.[86]

English was working in the hospital throughout this period, and, following her death in 1944, her obituary in the *East Galway Democrat* recorded that, during English's time there, 'Ballinasloe was the first mental hospital in Ireland to start electroconvulsive therapy.'[87]

Electroconvulsive therapy refers to the use of electricity, applied across the brain, to produce epileptic-type seizures (convulsions). Convulsive therapy was based on the idea that seizures were therapeutic in individuals with mental illness, and it built on the more general enthusiasm for biological treatments, such as insulin coma therapy, in the early twentieth century.[88] Insulin therapy had been introduced by Manfred Sakel, an Austrian psychiatrist and neurophysiologist, in the early 1930s and initially involved administering insulin to individuals with mental illness in order to increase weight and inhibit excitement.[89] Sakel noted, however, that the unintentional comas occasionally induced by insulin appeared to produce remission in schizophrenia. As a result, inducing coma was soon regarded as the key therapeutic mechanism of insulin amongst the mentally ill.

Some years later, programmes of convulsive therapy were introduced by Ladislas Joseph Meduna, a Hungarian neurologist who would, in 1938, go on to develop electroconvulsive therapy, with Ugo Cerletti, an Italian neurologist at the Rome University Psychiatric Clinic.[90] In the early years, however, seizures were induced using chemicals rather than electricity. Cardiazol was the trade-name of pentamethylenetetrazol, a camphor-like compound, used initially by Meduna for convulsive treatment of schizophrenia.[91] In 1935, Meduna reported positive results in ten out of the first twenty-six of his patients to receive Cardiazol treatment.[92] As a result, convulsive treatment soon spread to other psychiatric centres throughout Europe and beyond. The first recorded use of Cardiazol in England appears to have been at Moorcroft House, a private institution in Middlesex, in 1937. As the 1930s progressed, Cardiazol treatment became the most widely used physical treatment in public mental hospitals in Great Britain.[93]

In Ireland, physical treatments were also introduced throughout the 1930s. In July 1938, for example, Dr John Dunne introduced insulin coma therapy at Grangegorman Mental Hospital in Dublin.[94] Dunne reported that the first patient to receive the treatment, a 25-year-old woman, recovered sufficiently to return home. In 1950, Dunne published a relatively detailed, systematic analysis of insulin treatment at the hospital, reporting that 405 out of 605 patients treated with insulin had recovered.[95]

There is insufficient primary historical evidence to determine precisely when the focus of physical treatments moved from insulin coma to convulsive therapy in Irish asylums. As a result, it is not possible definitively to prove or disprove the assertion, in English's obituary in the *East Galway Democrat*, that 'Ballinasloe was the first mental hospital in Ireland to start electroconvulsive therapy.'[96]

It is clear, however, that Ballinasloe was, in a general sense, to the forefront of the introduction of novel therapies during English's time there. This was especially and demonstrably true in relation to convulsive therapy. In December 1939, the Committee of Management in Ballinasloe reported receiving a communication from the 'Local Government Department … stating that the Minister has no objection to the proposal to carry out Cardiazol treatment on certain patients provided the RMS accepts responsibility'.[97] The reference to Cardiazol in Ballinasloe in December 1939 is the earliest known reference to convulsive therapy in an Irish context, and occurred during English's time at the asylum.

Convulsive therapy was to soon move on from Cardiazol, however, and, in April 1942, Dunne introduced electroconvulsive therapy at Grangegorman Mental Hospital in Dublin.[98] Again, Dunne reported significant rates of recovery with electroconvulsive therapy, as 209 out of 327 patients with 'involutional melancholia' (depression) were recorded as 'recovered' following electroconvulsive therapy.[99]

This was a time of both deep therapeutic challenges and great therapeutic enthusiasm, especially for innovative treatments, in Irish asylums. In Ballinasloe, English, like Dunne, was to face many therapeutic challenges, including tuberculosis, which had become a substantial issue throughout all of Ireland's asylum system.[100] In 1913, English applied (unsuccessfully) for the post of 'Tuberculosis Officer for Roscommon'[101] and tuberculosis would duly become an especially challenging problem for English towards the end of her career (see below).

There were myriad other problems in the Ballinasloe hospital, too, including recurring instances of patients escaping from the institution. In 1933, the RMS, Mills, reported to the Committee of Management that one patient escaped from the hospital farm, where 'he took off his boots and ran "like a deer", leaving all his pursuers well behind. He was taken back later by the Guards'.[102] Mills 'was not blaming anybody for the patient's escape'. In 1940, another patient, a 'harmless man, between 30 and 35 years of age … got away from the dining hall on the occasion of a weekly dance'.[103] The RMS described the man as 'a very active and intelligent patient' and the patient proved duly difficult to locate.

Some of those who escaped died by suicide. In 1939, there was a 'sworn Inquiry' into the suicide of a female patient, who was committed to the hospital on 21 December 1938 and whose body was recovered from the nearby River Suck on 22 July 1939.[104] According to Lyons, RMS, this 'patient suffered from melancholia', 'had suicidal tendencies', and had 'been under supervision since her admission'. English, as 'assistant medical officer', gave evidence to the Inquiry:

> I am in charge of the Female Division. I knew deceased. She was a potential suicide and nurses were provided with suicidal caution cards in her case. I never saw evidence of a desire on the part of the patient to commit suicide whilst she was under my care. She was very depressed and was anxious to go home.[105]

English was questioned about how this suicidal patient could escape from the asylum grounds:

> I never knew of any patient escaping at the place where this patient escaped. The wall was raised five or six years ago. Benches are not placed close to the wall. A patient escaped over boundary wall more than five years ago, but no patient has previously escaped since the wall was raised. This patient was in suicidal division, all of whom (fifty-eight) were potential suicides. These patients were under constant supervision. The wall is eight or ten feet high. There was an upright stake near where patient climbed on to wall; this may have been used by patient to climb the wall. The stake has now been removed.[106]

Regarding nursing supervision, Mrs O'Connor, 'acting assistant matron', stated that there were three nurses 'in charge of fifty-eight patients' and, while she 'would like more than three nurses' she was nonetheless 'satisfied with number of nurses on ground'. The Inquiry concluded that while 'no blame attaches to any of the nurses', there should be 'at least one nurse or attendant to every fourteen or fifteen patients and that the group should be under the constant supervision of all the staff allotted to their care'.[107]

This was not a new problem, a similar Inquiry into a patient suicide in 1927 concluded 'that the division which the patient occupied is not sufficiently staffed' and 'where the lives or the safety of the patients is at stake it is false economy to reduce the numbers of the staff below the margin of safety'.[108]

English took her therapeutic enthusiasms well beyond the hospital walls, with a strong focus on population health and wellbeing. She served as honorary secretary of the Ballinasloe branch of the Women's National Health Association (WNHA), the first branch to be established in county Galway, on 18 March 1908.[109] The WNHA had been founded in 1907 by Lady Aberdeen with the initial aim of addressing tuberculosis and infant mortality. Lady Clonbrock, a campaigning Unionist and wife of the lord lieutenant of the county, was president of the Ballinasloe branch while English was honorary secretary; this may account for why English's name appears in just one report from the Ballinasloe branch during this period.[110] The branch was nonetheless an active one, inviting pioneering veterinary surgeon Aleen Cust to deliver a lecture to the branch.

In addition to her involvement in the WNHA, English had various other involvements outside of the hospital including, for example, organizing Red Cross lectures in Ballinasloe during the two World Wars.[111] As a result of these activities, as well as her position at the mental hospital and political involvement, English became well known in Ballinasloe and the surrounding area.

One local man remembers meeting English frequently when he was aged between twelve and fourteen years and English was in her sixties.[112] Like many locals, he referred to English as 'Lady English' owing to her dignified bearing and the respect she commanded in the area. English would be out in her horse and trap, driven by a patient, and would stop and talk with the young boy for up to twenty minutes when she met him on the road. He remembers English as being of light build, invariably well wrapped-up and always accompanied by dogs. English insisted that they both speak in Irish. English took a particular interest in the boy's schooling, teachers, and family life. English would praise his use of Irish and bid him farewell with a cheerful 'Beannacht Leat!'[113]

Further Challenges in the Mental Hospital

During the 1920s and 1930s the Ballinasloe mental hospital continued to expand. In 1924 a new building, The Pines, was acquired.[114] The Pines was formerly St Joseph's College, where English's friend, Bishop Dignan, had served as president from 1904 to 1919.[115] After it became part of the mental hospital, The Pines accommodated 140 patients. There was still substantial pressure on beds, however, and in 1929, the hospital engineer submitted proposals for remodelling four workhouses to make them suitable as 'auxiliary asylums' in Portumna (260 patients, at a cost of £22,000), Castlerea (70 patients, £21,000), Boyle (250 patients, £22,000) and Strokestown (230 patients, £27,000).[116]

There were also developments proposed for Ballinasloe and agreed in 1933, at a cost of £255,000. These buildings were occupied in 1939 and included several new wards (accommodating 410 patients) and a Nurse's Home (accommodating sixty-three nurses) as well as recreation rooms and lecture facilities.[117]

Life in the hospital was difficult, as it was in most mental hospitals at this time. There were constant problems with overcrowding leading to myriad difficulties managing large numbers of patients in constricted environments. At a meeting of the Ballinasloe Asylum Committee in April 1916, 'the report of the Lunacy Inspectors on their recent inspection of the institution was read':

> It stated that the patients in some of the male and female divisions were huddled together, practically naked, in a cold ward, lying on wet straw, and the condition of things was scandalous. They did not think that in any civilised country such a condition of things existed as they found in the wards visited. It was hard to realise that creatures who could neither speak nor act for themselves would be left in such a manner.[118]

The Chairman described it as a 'very strong report' and the Committee sought to establish 'who was responsible for the awful state of things. The Clerk said that Dr Kirwan, RMS (who was in the RAMC) [Royal Army Medical Corps] had said that it would take £3 nightly to keep clothes on the patients and furniture in the divisions referred to'. English, who was acting RMS in Kirwan's absence, 'said that she was not aware that the patients were treated in the manner stated,' and it was agreed that immediate action would be taken.

Owing in large part to these overcrowded, unsanitary conditions, death rates in the Irish asylums were high, with many deaths attributable to infectious diseases – diphtheria,[119] typhoid,[120] influenza[121] – amongst other causes, including acts of violence.[122] In November 1928, a female patient in Ballinasloe 'was charged with the murder of another inmate' and found to be 'insane and incapable of pleading. She was ordered to be detained in a criminal lunatic asylum during the pleasure of the Governor-General of the Free State' (i.e. indefinitely).[123]

Hospital staff were also at risk of illness and injury. In 1929, the Committee of Management received a letter from the Department of Local Government and Public Health enquiring in some detail about steps taken following the death of a nurse who suffered from diphtheria.[124] Also in 1929, the RMS, Mills, reported that English was absent from the January meeting of the Committee of Management because she 'has been laid up with an attack of illness. I will require a substitute for her'.[125] In 1930, English's colleague 'Dr Delaney sustained a severe sprain of the leg by being knocked down on the stairs … by a patient who was trying to escape.'[126]

Management of disturbed patients presented a real challenge. In 1929, the RMS, Mills, reported to the Committee of Management that 'a patient in No. 9 suicidal division damaged a padded cell and I hold the attendants in charge responsible. The house is very much overcrowded'.[127] The patient had damaged the padded cell using a small religious medal. Mills was away at the time and English told the Committee 'that it would be almost impossible to find out where the patient got the medal. The night men assured her [English] that he had not got the medal at night and suggested that someone might have dropped it at breakfast time'.[128] The attendants involved were fined £1 each.

During this period there were also industrial relations problems at many Irish mental hospitals, including Ballinasloe. In 1918, attendants at Monaghan Asylum had gone on strike demanding improved pay and union recognition, and achieved moderate concessions from management.[129] In early January 1919, however, the Monaghan dispute escalated and asylum staff occupied the asylum. Dramatically, the red flag was raised over the asylum and the Monaghan Asylum Soviet came into being. These assertive actions produced significant results by securing improvements in both pay and hours, and, perhaps more importantly, setting an example for similar institutions throughout Ireland and Britain.

In Ireland, at least some of these industrial relations problems found their roots in 'a series of "trade-offs" between priorities' as efforts to establish the new Irish state during the early 1900s 'resulted in a diminishing of earlier initiatives related to training and ultimately in a prolonged period of retrenchment' for asylum workers.[130] In essence, the early phases of national autonomy in Ireland led to sacrifices as part of the progressive realisation of self-governance, and one of these sacrifices was timely improvement in training and conditions for asylum workers.

In July 1923, staff at the Ballinasloe Mental Hospital presented an 'ultimatum' to the Committee of Management 'threatening that they will go out on strike' if 'certain demands are not favourably considered'.[131] The Committee was not entirely convinced by all of the claims, however, as 'the Most Rev Dr O'Doherty, Bishop of Clonfert, who presided, characterised as preposterous the claim for fires at 5pm in the present warm weather, and this claim was unanimously turned down'. Overall, however, most of the claims seemed reasonable and were 'favourably considered'.

Sustained industrial peace proved elusive, however, and by September 1924 staff in Ballinasloe were out on strike and 'about fifty Civic Guards' especially requisitioned for night duty at the hospital.[132] In this case, 'the trouble arose through the appointment of a back gate porter who was not a member of the Mental Hospital Attendants' Union'.[133] As a result, the attendants went out on strike:

Dr Mills, resident medical superintendent … described the scenes of confusion which followed the departure of the attendants, who took the keys of cells with them, and said the strikers ill-treated other attendants who refused to go with them. Before they all left some of the attendants opened the cells of the suicidal and homicidal patients and allowed them to escape into the corridors of the institution. Two other patients escaped, and two female attendants dragged an epileptic patient down the hall and tried to force her into the matron's rooms.

He (Dr Mills) and Dr Ada English assisted by his wife and family, including a very young boy, and the depleted staff, tried to manage until the evening when he found that the telephone wires were cut in two places, and that he could not telephone for assistance. Pandemonium reigned throughout the asylum, and at night, fearing for the lives of many of the patients, he requested the strikers to return, sending the gate porter, over whose appointment the strike took place, away.[134]

As a result, 'the gate porter, whose appointment was the cause of the strike, decided at midnight on Saturday to relinquish the post, and was escorted from the building by Civic Guards, after which the strikers entered the institution and resumed duty'.[135]

Industrial relations continued to present challenges throughout the 1930s[136] and in 1938 employees in mental hospitals, at their conference in Mullingar, demanded 'the general establishment of the forty-eight-hour week, three weeks' annual leave, and an increase of twenty per cent in existing salaries'.[137] One delegate from Ballinasloe, Mr M. Kelly, drew attention to retirement arrangements, stating that 'retirement after twenty-five years' service should be compulsory. How many at the age of sixty or sixty-five years were able to deal with a violent patient, escapes, or do duty in a tuberculosis ward?'

By this time, however, industrial relations problems were a staple feature of hospital life, and they soon faced stiff competition for the attention of the Committee of Management in Ballinasloe because a new and arguably more serious problem emerged in the late 1930s and was to occupy the attention of the Committee for several months, leading, ultimately, to the Committee's demise.

Selection of a New Resident Medical Superintendent

In 1935, Mills, the much-loved RMS, was taken ill and English, as acting RMS, attended Committee meetings in his place. On 6 November 1935, she reported on Mills's absence:

I very much regret having to report that Dr Mills is absent in hospital and will probably not be back for a few weeks… I am certain I am only voicing the feelings of you all when I say that we hope and pray for his speedy recovery. Dr Mills has always been courteous and obliging to every member of the Committee. His zeal and devotion to the interests of the patients, his kindness to and consideration for the staff, one and all, is beyond reproach. As a medical man he is second to none… Personally, I am very sorry that anything should be the matter with such a painstaking and capable official.[138]

English was, however, a worthy temporary replacement and, following the first Committee meeting in Mills's absence, Committee members 'proposed a vote of congratulation to Dr English on the able manner in which she had conducted the business of the meeting' and 'the resolution was passed with general acclaim'.[139]

On 18 March 1936, Mills died in a Dublin hospital, following a prolonged illness.[140] He had been originally appointed to the asylum in Ballinasloe in May 1893 and been RMS since 1916. His obituary in the *Connacht Tribune* reflected genuine sadness at his loss:

[Mills] took a very deep interest in his work and as an executive officer and medical man he was recognised as second to none in Ireland. Since 1916, when he was appointed RMS his work and research on behalf of the insane have been of valuable assistance in the care and treatment of insanity. He often paid a visit to the English and Scottish, as well as the mental institutions in other parts of Ireland, and his experience and the knowledge gained were always placed at the disposal of his committee to whom he was continually making new recommendations for the treatment of his charges in Ballinasloe… The care of the patients was his one absorbing thought – how they were to be better housed especially – and no more fitting tribute could be paid to his work than that of a former chairman who said publicly on one occasion that Dr Mills knew everyone of his 2,000 patients there individually and by name … he could tell each of them by the peculiarity of their manners and ways; he knew them all and the patients had always a deep respect for him… [He] took a personal interest in all the members of his staff, made the several appointments in the institution always in their best interests, and especially in the better interests of the patients and the discipline of the house… He was recognised as an able lecturer in the treatment of insanity and was nearly always present in the lecture hall where he conducted the classes in the institution and thus built up an efficient and qualified staff of nurses and attendants.[141]

Following the death of Mills, the Committee of Management nominated English for the post of RMS but the Local Appointments Commissioners gave the position to Dr Bernard Lyons, who had qualified in medicine from the National University of Ireland in 1918 and worked in the mental hospital in Enniscorthy, County Wexford.

The decision to appoint Lyons caused consternation in Ballinasloe. By that time English had been working at the Ballinasloe Hospital for some thirty-two years and was well liked both locally and by the Committee of Management. Ballinasloe Urban Council wrote to the Department of Local Government and Public Health demanding an enquiry into the appointment of Lyons 'and the rejection of the application by Dr English, who had satisfactorily filled the position during the War years and since the death of Dr Mills'.[142]

At a meeting of the Committee of Management on 9 November 1936, English, acting RMS, read a stern letter from the Department of Local Government and Public Health 'stating that the Committee had failed to discharge a statutory duty which devolved on them to appoint Dr Lyons and that Dr Lyons was entitled to appointment from the date of the recommendation of the Local Appointment Commissioners, and that the appointment should be made without further delay'.[143] The Committee refused. One member pointed out that advertisement had indicated the 'person appointed must have a competent knowledge of Irish', and asked: 'What qualifications did Dr Lyons possess which Dr English did not, and which would counteract the knowledge of Irish which she has and he has not?' The Committee sent a resolution to this effect to the Department of Local Government and Public Health, refusing to make the appointment.

This controversy led to considerable complexity at the Department, not least because there was already difficulty regarding an appointment at the mental hospitals in Grangegorman and Portrane in Dublin.[144] Against this background, on 28 November 1936, three weeks after the meeting of the Ballinasloe Committee, Mr E.P. McCarron, secretary to the Department of Local Government and Public Health was abruptly removed from office. McCarron asked the Minister, Deputy Sean T. O'Kelly (Minister for Local Government and Public Health, 1932–39), why he had been removed and the Minister reportedly responded that the proceedings of the Committee at Grangegorman 'were a cause of embarrassment to him, having regard to political difficulties he had experienced over the filling of a vacancy in the post of resident medical superintendent at Ballinasloe and the candidature there of Dr Ada English'.[145]

McCarron tried to reassure the Minister that the issues were different in the two institutions: the issue in Grangegorman referred to its deputy RMS, a position which existed only in Grangegorman because Grangegorman was the only mental hospital in the country to have an auxiliary asylum (in Portrane). On the retirement of the RMS there, the *title* of the deputy RMS was changed to RMS, but the substantive *position* of RMS would be substantively filled in due course through the Local Appointments Commissioners (i.e. the same procedure as in Ballinasloe). In Ballinasloe, by contrast, 'Dr English was the assistant medical officer and not the deputy resident medical superintendent of the mental hospital and was a candidate for the vacant position there of resident medical superintendent.'[146]

McCarron was removed and the Department of Local Government and Public Health insisted on the appointment of Lyons in Ballinasloe. It may be significant that Minister O'Kelly had, like English, been a member of Sinn Féin and opposed to the Anglo-Irish Treaty. He later, however, joined de Valera in his newly-created political party, Fianna Fáil, and arguably compromised his position on the Treaty by becoming a member of Dáil Éireann. He later also served as president of Ireland (1945–59). English, by contrast, remained strongly anti-Treaty and unconvinced by the legitimacy of Dáil Éireann.[147]

In any case, in February 1937 the Committee in Ballinasloe was informed of the Department's insistence that 'when a recommendation has been made by the Local Appointments Commissioners it is obligatory on the Local Authority to appoint the person recommended' (i.e. Lyons).[148] If the Committee did not comply, the Department would 'institute proceedings by way of mandamus' and 'members of the Committee who, by their action, render themselves responsible for the proceedings would be named as special defendants and therefore liable for any costs incurred'. This startled and annoyed the Committee. One member stated: 'This is a threat.' Another responded: 'Terrible and immediate war!' A third was stoic: 'There is no way out but to obey.'

It transpired that the Local Appointments Commissioners had given Lyons three years in which to qualify in the Irish language, leading another Committee member to bemoan the government's lack of consistent or coherent emphasis on Irish, and announce that 'the Government is a fraud'. She was ruled out of order but, not a whit abashed, went on to suggest Lyons was appointed 'because he was a man'.

Another Committee member, Mr Colleran, concluded that 'the root of the disease is the Appointments Commissioners and the remedy is to get them abolished'. Another member, Mr Lambert, drew the Committee's attention to Dáil proceedings relevant to the topic:

We all regret very much that we were not able to press our recommendation of Dr English to success. One thing I resent very much is the statement of Deputy McDermott of Roscommon in the Dáil. Deputy McDermott suggested that we were out to take the candidate by the throat and take his position for Dr English. He is wrong. Dr English never relied on her national record, outstanding as it is. She relied on long and valued service and experience. She conducted the duties entrusted to her with credit to herself and to the institution. I regret that we had Galway deputies in the Dáil and that they allowed Deputy McDermott of Roscommon to refer to Dr English as Salome demanding the head of Mr McCarron from Herod de Valera.[149]

In the Dáil on 3 February 1937, Mr John A. Costello, a Fine Gael deputy, had called for a 'select committee' to 'be set up, publicly to investigate and report to the Dáil on all the facts and circumstances connected with and surrounding the decision of the Executive Council that the retention of Mr E.P. McCarron in his post of Secretary to the Department of Local Government and Public Health was no longer possible'.[150] Costello linked his request with events in Ballinasloe:

It is a matter of common notoriety that so far as any intimation has been given by the Government of the reasons why they removed Mr McCarron from office, that those reasons were in some way or another connected with an appointment which had been made in the Portrane asylum and had some connection with some events in connection with Ballinasloe asylum. It is a matter that everybody is aware of that a vacancy occurred in the position of resident medical superintendent of the Ballinasloe Mental Home some short time ago through the death of Dr Mills, the then resident medical superintendent. In accordance with the settled practice of the Department of Local Government, that post fell to be filled through the machinery of the Local Appointments Commissioners, and intimation was conveyed to the committee administering the affairs of the Ballinasloe Mental Home that the Minister could not accede to the request which had been put forward that a certain medical officer who then held a position in the mental home should be promoted to the position of resident medical superintendent. It is well known that the greatest possible influence was brought to bear upon the Minister and the Government by the Party from which the Government is formed to secure the appointment of a particular individual to that post.[151]

Deputy Frank McDermott of Roscommon, a member of the Centre Party, nominated by the Taoiseach, added colour to the debate:

> The present Government are at least singularly unlucky on this occasion if their conduct has been as virtuous as they claim it has been, because it is within common knowledge that there was a fierce agitation against the Department of Local Government, and inferentially against Mr McCarron in particular, as its permanent head, over the Ballinasloe appointment. Superficially, what we see is this: we see Salome, in the person of Doctor Ada English, demanding from King Herod, in the person of the Minister for Local Government, the head of John the Baptist – in the person of the unfortunate Mr McCarron – on a charger. That is what it is apt to look like to the general public, and there is a danger of civil servants getting the impression that they will be sacrificed, if the Government finds itself in a tight place, in order to appease the supporters of the Government.[152]

The Dáil voted on Deputy Costello's request for a 'select committee' to investigate McCarron's removal and it was soundly defeated by sixty-one votes to forty-four. The following week, the Chairman of the Committee of Management of the Ballinasloe Mental Hospital, Mr Mark Killilea TD, a Fianna Fáil Dáil deputy, told the Committee that if he had been in the Dáil for that debate McDermott 'would not have been allowed to pass with that, but we don't sit there idly listening to all the foolish talk that goes on'.[153] In line with the rest of the Committee, Killilea still maintained that that 'all of us are as anxious to have Dr English' as RMS, but the battle was now lost and Lyons was duly appointed to the post. Predictably, there was significant consternation when it became known that Lyons, as opposed to English, had been appointed.[154]

On 8 March 1937 English reported to the Committee that Lyons had visited the hospital but found that the 'late RMS's house was in a bad state of repair and he could not think of transferring his family there'.[155] Even on this issue, the bickering between the Committee in Ballinasloe and the Department of Local Government and Public Health continued: the Committee initially allowed £1,500 for a new house for the RMS but then 'the architect, Mr B. Barrett, wrote that he was told unofficially that the Minister for Local Government was willing to allow up to £2,500 for this purpose'.[156] Miss Ashe, a Committee member who had previously spoken strongly in support of English, was not at all impressed with this inflated amount for Lyons's house, commenting that 'a house costing £1,500 was good enough for anyone'.

This matter rumbled on for several months. In May 1937, English reported to the Committee that 'Dr Lyons was not willing to take up duty until the residence was ready for him. She had asked if he would come in as soon as two rooms were ready but he would not approve of that.'[157] Lyons finally took up his post on 15 June 1937 and, at his first Committee meeting, the issue of his new residence was again raised, not least because the cost had now climbed to £2,800.[158] Lyons expressed a preference that the house be located with the asylum boundaries so 'it would be easier for me to keep supervision over the place'. Miss Ashe, ever sceptical, noted that even 'if the doctor is here today he may not be here next year'. It took longer than a single year, but Miss Ashe's words about Lyons's future would ultimately prove prophetic.

A 'Sworn Inquiry' at Ballinasloe Mental Hospital (1940)

Two years after Lyons's arrival in Ballinasloe, on 10 July 1939, there was a dramatic meeting of the Committee of Management of Ballinasloe Mental Hospital at which the Committee 'unanimously decided to ask the Minister to hold a Public Sworn Inquiry into the management of the whole institution since 1934, when the present Committee took office'.[159] At the next meeting, on 14 August 1939, a more detailed but equally dramatic resolution was passed:

> That the Committee of Management desire to have the following matters investigated by Public Sworn Inquiry:-
>
> (1) That the public have got an impression as a result of the publications in the Press from time to time that this Institution has not been properly run, and that the patients have been neglected as a result.
> (2) That the RMS has from time to time made statements to the effect that he found the place in a mess.
> (3) That the Local Government Department has held private enquiries, of which the Committee were not aware, into certain matters in connection with the management of the Institution.
> (4) That there is and has been a lack of harmony amongst the Officers of the Institution.[160]

The calls for an Inquiry stemmed from a long-standing 'difference of opinion between the medical staff and a controversy between the RMS, Dr Bernard Lyons, and the Administrator, the Rev E. Hughes, Ballinasloe regarding the latter's authority for his visit to the hospital in an endeavour to adjust existing differences some time ago'.[161] At a meeting of the Committee of Management of Ballinasloe Mental Hospital in July 1939, Hughes 'read letters from the Department [of Local Government and Public Health] and the Inspector for Mental Hospitals, which, he said, gave him authority to go into the institution'.

Lyons stated that 'on making inquiries in the Department he was told that Father Hughes had no authority to come to the institution'. Lyons 'alleged that Father Hughes told him that if there was not harmony created in the place the RMS [Lyons] would have to go'.[162]

This kind of dispute was not unique to Ballinasloe, as the power of doctors was continually contested and debated since the foundation of the asylums in the 1800s.[163] This dispute appeared especially bitter however, as Hughes dismissed Lyons's allegation as a 'concoction' and demanded an apology, which Lyons refused to give.[164] The Chairman, Mr Mark Killilea, TD, noted that 'the Committee was a long time trying to adjust the differences between the doctors and failed'. He proposed that a sworn Inquiry be held and others agreed, with Mr Beegan TD, adding 'that there was no trouble there until Dr Lyons, RMS, came'. Lyons responded 'that the place was in a "rotten mess" when he came there. He had to do his best to clean it up, but the trouble was still going on.'[165] In the end, 'the Chairman said that the thing had already got a good deal of publicity, and the sworn inquiry was the only way to settle the existing differences. The Committee were unanimous in asking for the inquiry.'

The *Irish Times* reported the Committee's call for an inquiry in some detail:

> The Chairman, Mr M. Killalea, TD, said there was a lot of talk going around and with the publication in the Press, it was only right and desirable that there should be an inquiry and have everything above board. Since 1934 there was a general impression abroad that the place was in a 'mess,' and this impression should be cleared up… Dr Ada English, Acting RMS, said that the doctors welcomed the inquiry. It would give them a chance of clearing up their part in it and she believed that the Chairman had a letter from the Department concerning the matter.[166]

The 'Sworn Inquiry was held … on the 3rd, 4th and 5th January [1940] into the management of the Institution' since 1934,[167] and it also had regard to 'unfavourable press reports re administration etc. and lack of harmony between officers of institution'.[168] English both gave evidence herself and was represented legally by Mr A.F. Comyn, BA, a Ballinasloe solicitor.[169] The inquiry was conducted by Dr R.P. McDonnell, Chief Medical Inspector to the Department of Local Government and Public Health.[170]

The Inspector noted at the outset that 'it's very hard to know how to hold an inquiry unless you know what to inquire into'.[171] He was not at all impressed with what he found in the Ballinasloe hospital:

> There was a lot of little petty squabbles amongst officials. This, I think, the Committee of Management should have settled themselves. We cannot send

down an Inspector here to hold an inquiry into every time these officials have differences... This is one long series of small petty squabbles which should never be the subject of an inquiry. We will endeavour to smooth out some of these things, and I have the assistance of some very distinguished legal gentlemen, and they will help me to disentangle some of these.[172]

The inquiry then heard evidence of newspaper coverage of mental hospital affairs and, in particular, reports that 'it has been referred to on more than one occasion by the RMS [Lyons] that he found the place in a "mess".'[173] The inquiry also heard from English, that, on 4 February 1939, she had written to the Department of Local Government and Public Health stating that, at a recent meeting, 'several allegations were made by the RMS about the medical staff in general and myself in particular'.[174] It was 'very disturbing to me to have aspersions made on my truthfulness, and on the manner in which I carry out my work,' and 'apart from the injustice involved, it obviously undermines seriously the discipline of the institution and the welfare of the patients'.[175] It did not rest easy with English that she felt compelled to write such a letter: 'I dislike intensely having to do this, but the whole position is getting intolerable.'[176]

English went on to specify the allegations made against her:

I will not worry you reciting events leading up to this. You are already aware of them, but arising out of what might have been a friendly discussion and arrangement of work, etc., Dr Lyons made the most sweeping allegations. 'The doctors here do the very minimum amount of work.' 'If they are wanted, you have to send for them.' 'If I went around the hospital a hundred times a month, I would never see one of them on duty,' and again 'I say that the doctors are doing the very minimum work.' Later on there was a reference to your [the Inspector's] visit here and to the question as to whether I should have had three calendar months['] leave last year. Dr Lyons's comment on this was: 'You told the Inspector that you got three calendar months. The letter from the Department was produced and it put the lie down your throat'.... As you were there, sir, you yourself can judge the appropriateness of this remark. You can see, Mr Inspector, from these extracts that the position is intolerable, and, in order to avoid seeking other measures to protect myself, I am bringing the matter before you and the Department and request that some action be taken to prevent the continuation of this conduct. I would welcome, if it should be necessary, a sworn Inquiry into the manner in which I have discharged my duties. Obviously, if Dr Lyons is right, I should be dismissed and if he is wrong I should at least be vindicated. I may mention that I asked Dr Lyons, before the meeting, to settle the matter between ourselves but he refused. Furthermore, I asked him the following day would he apologise before I would have to take further steps in the matter, and he again refused.[177]

Killilea, as Chairman of the Committee of Management, gave evidence that the 'lack of harmony' was basically 'Dr Lyons versus the others'.[178] Killilea confirmed that he had heard Lyons make statements that English quoted in her letter.[179] However, the Committee of Management was unable to establish the veracity or otherwise of these statements: 'The Committee were in a helpless position. One doctor said one thing and another said another ... That is why we asked for a sworn inquiry.'[180]

At this point, the Inspector noted that 'up to now, we have no proof or evidence except the statement of the RMS that the assistant medical officers were not doing their work. We have no sworn testimony that the lady and gentleman were not doing their work. So for the moment we have to move on that statement as made and has not been proved.'[181]

As the inquiry examined these matters in greater depth, it became apparent that differences of opinion between staff members stemmed from a diversity of sources. It appears, for example that Lyons sought to introduce a formal roster system for doctors, but that the doctors 'suggested it should be left as it was, that from time to time and from day to day the doctors should work it out amongst themselves'.[182] Interestingly, English was not among the doctors who voiced objections to Lyons's proposals at that time, even though she was not enthusiastic about them.[183]

English, in her evidence, was clear in her view that Lyons's alleged comments about her amounted to an accusation that she had neglected her duty and were 'a reflection on my professional career. It was repeated and elaborated on that I was never to be seen if he went around the house one hundred times a month'.[184] She asserted strongly that 'I have done my work, whether satisfactory to Dr Lyons or not.'[185]

Regarding her alleged untruthfulness, English stated that she 'was away on leave. Somebody wrote and said that I was granted three months['] leave. I took it that meant three calendar months. I had a letter from Dr Lyons calling me back at the end of twelve weeks. I felt a bit sore about it...'[186] English did return from leave, but not before calling in to the Inspector (who, by coincidence, was now conducting the Inquiry) to ask 'if I only got three lunar months'.[187] The Inspector promised to find out. English returned to work, as requested by Lyons:

I came back fully intend[ing] to ask for another week as I considered that I was done out of a week. When I came back I found a fresh row on. I think Dr Delaney was reported for creating discord on the female side of the house. When I found a fresh row on (there were rows every other day) I did not want to start another one, so I said I would let it slide.[188]

English went on to allege that Lyons, at a meeting on 9 July 1939, intimated that English had lied about her leave and had, in November 1938, made a similar statement.[189] English also said that while she hadn't actually voiced an objection to Lyons's proposal for new rosters, she 'thought it was a mistake'.[190] The Inspector, in search of hard evidence, was unimpressed: 'We cannot investigate your thoughts.'[191]

In a spirited interchange, English was cross-examined on the necessity for a new RMS, such as Lyons, to make these kinds of changes to the way an institution is run:

> Mr Cecil Lavery, KC (appearing for Lyons): There is no use in having an RMS unless he makes some improvements.
> English: We have learned that.
> Lavery: A new broom sweeps clean.
> English: It sometimes sweeps out valuables.
> Lavery: The RMS must prevail.
> English: Precisely: the heavy artillery.[192]

As the inquiry wore on, it transpired that a letter had been sent from the Department of Local Government and Public Health to the Chairman of the Committee of Management of Ballinasloe Mental Hospital on 12 June 1939, some months prior to the inquiry, stating that 'the Minister is satisfied that Dr English is discharging her duties effectively and well, and at all times is solicitous to the welfare of patients under her care'.[193] English had hinted at the existence of such a letter prior to the inquiry[194] but it appears that the Chairman of the Committee did not read this letter in public at a Committee meeting, possibly because the envelope may have been marked 'personal'.[195] It appears that the contents of this letter were only made public during the inquiry; had the letter's contents been made public earlier, the entire inquiry might well have been avoided.[196]

In any case, the inquiry dragged on at some length, with 'Dr John Delaney, medical officer' outlining a disagreement he had with Lyons, and considerable attention subsequently devoted to the question of whether or not one or both of the two doctors was under the influence of alcohol at the time.[197] The inquiry also heard evidence from 'Mrs Nora Harris-O'Connor, Matron' regarding various other related matters including a suggestion (never proven) that she had been absent without notifying the RMS.[198]

Lyons, in his evidence, provided a clear and robust account of his statements,[199] admitting he had stated that he found the hospital in a 'rotten mess' when he arrived there,[200] but specifying that when he used the phrase 'rotten mess' he was referring only to the matter of a land steward who was, he said, 'sent to jail for stealing cattle'.[201] Lyons also presented a series of observations to support his statement that the 'doctors were doing the very minimum amount of work', noting, for example, that 'I never got a report of a surprise night visit by a doctor.'[202] In addition, 'I never saw a doctor on the lands. I said if I was round the grounds 100 times a month I would not see a doctor.'[203] Nonetheless, Lyons stated that he had never charged any of the doctors with specific neglect of duty, but rather stated more generally that they 'were doing the very minimum amount of work' in an overall sense.[204]

Lyons also presented a series of observations to support his concerns about the level of competence among nursing staff.[205] He stated, *inter alia*, that when he arrived in Ballinasloe in June 1937[206] he found that 'the patients' filthy clothing was rinsed out' in 'the baths in which the patients would be bathed in afterwards' and 'the way the food was handed out to the patients you would think they were a lot of savages'.[207] On the issue of who might be responsible for this state of affairs at the time of Lyons's arrival, the Inspector was clear that 'the Committee was primarily responsible for having it like that. They should have seen that it was not like that'.[208] Asked if the institution was still a 'mess', Lyons replied that it was 'improving'.[209] With regard to the serving of food, English testified that matters were indeed now much improved.[210]

Regarding the dispute about English's three months of leave, Lyons admitted saying 'I had to go down to the office and get the letter to put the lie down your throat,' but added that 'only for I was a wee bit hot I would not have said it'.[211] Lyons stated he regretted the words although, on cross-examination, it was pointed out that he had repeated his words at a later date, 'in the presence of the press'.[212] Nonetheless, Lyons clearly regretted his words and, on further cross-examination, also acknowledged that English 'has done a certain amount of visits at night'.[213]

Regarding the question of English's leave, the Inspector provided a definitive answer: 'Dr English was told in the Department that she got three calendar months. I can swear to that I told her.'[214] For his part, Lyons stated that there had simply been a 'misunderstanding over the letter'.[215] He withdrew 'absolutely' his accusation that English had lied[216] and said he 'would rather have used nicer words when speaking to a lady'.[217] Asked if he agreed 'with the Department's letter to the Chairman that Dr English discharges her duties efficiently', Lyons was unambiguous: 'I do'.[218]

Some cross-examinations were notably heated, and occasionally revealed a great deal about internal hospital politics:

> Mr Bradford England (appearing for the Matron): Would I be right in saying that when on the rounds you walk with the Head Nurse in front, instead of walking with the Matron or Dr English?
> Lyons: Yes.
> England: Would it not be better to walk with the Matron?
> Lyons: The Matron and Dr English are often behind us. I go quickly.
> England: You made certain charges against Dr English; was not a letter vindicating her submitted here?
> Lyons: I made no charge against Dr English.
> England: You made charges against the doctors here.
> Lyons: I made no charges.
> England: I am suggesting to you that your conduct here is not extraordinary considering your long association with lunatics.
> Inspector: That is not so. I will not allow that.[219]

The inquiry was completed on 5 January 1940 and matters were tense while an outcome was awaited. At the Committee meeting of 11 March 1940, Delaney, assistant medical officer, was ordered to leave the meeting for allegedly 'prompting some members at the end of the table and criticising other members remarks'.[220] One member said he believed that there was 'an order made some time ago' that 'no other doctor be allowed to take part in the committee's discussion but the RMS'. One Committee member described this as 'tyranny' and Delaney asked: 'Why should I be asked to retire? What have I done wrong?' Nonetheless, Delaney withdrew from the meeting.

The outcome to the inquiry became known on 11 June 1940 when Dr Joseph Kearney, of Herbert Park, Dublin, received a letter from the Department of Local Government and Public Health 'advising the Commissioner [i.e. Kearney] of the dissolution of the Committee [of Management of Ballinasloe Mental Hospital], and enclosing Sealed Order appointing him to administer the affairs of the Institution, and transferring to him the several powers, duties and property of the Joint Committee of Management'.[221] The Committee was thus dissolved.

Kearney held his first meeting as Commissioner on 14 June 1940. The only other people present were 'Doctors B. Lyons, A. English, J. Delaney, and the Matron'.[222] The Minutes of the Committee of Management over previous months record that English had two periods of sick leave in the months leading up to this meeting (29 December 1939 to 13 January 1940, and 1 February

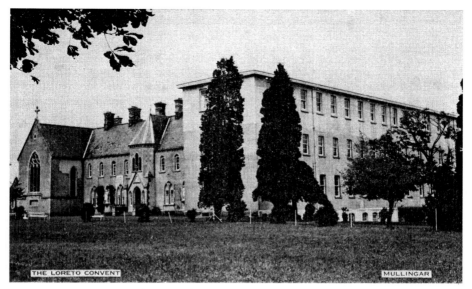

1. Loreto Convent, Longford Road, Mullingar, Co Westmeath, where English attended for her secondary schooling.

Source: © National Inventory of Architectural Heritage. Used with permission.

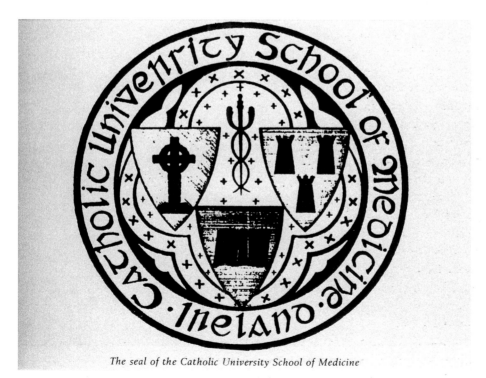

The seal of the Catholic University School of Medicine

2. The Seal of the Catholic University School of Medicine, where English pursued her medical studies, graduating from the Royal University in 1903.

Source: Meenan, F.O.C., *Cecilia Street: The Catholic University School of Medicine, 1855-1931* (Dublin: Gill and Macmillan, 1987). Used with permission..

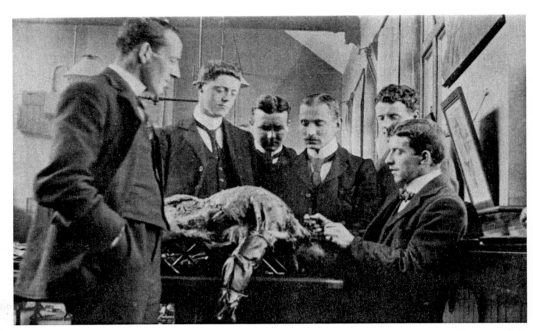

3. The Dissecting Room at the Catholic University School of Medicine c.1900, where English attended.

Source: Meenan, F.O.C., *Cecilia Street: The Catholic University School of Medicine, 1855-1931* (Dublin: Gill and Macmillan, 1987). Used with permission.

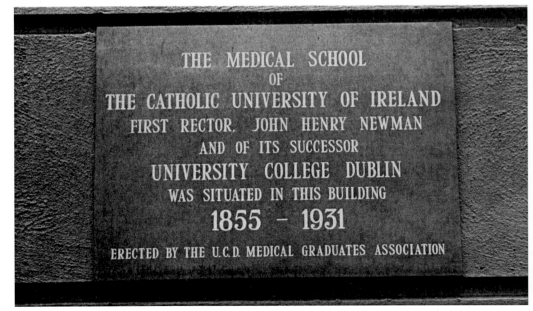

4. Plaque on the restored building in Cecilia Street which originally housed the Medical School Ada English attended.

Source: Meenan, F.O.C., *Cecilia Street: The Catholic University School of Medicine, 1855-1931* (Dublin: Gill and Macmillan, 1987). Used with permission.

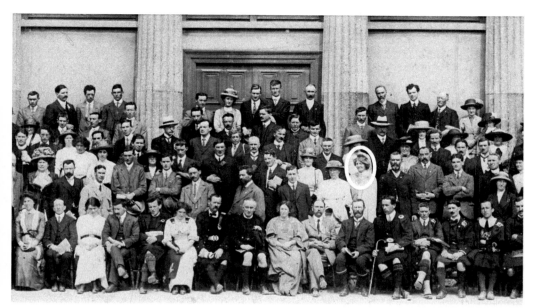

5. English, photographed attending a Gaelic League national convention in Galway in 1913. English (with no hat) is in the second row from the front, beside Máire Ní Chinnéide (with hat) and behind Eoin McNeill (seated in the front row, holding a book). Douglas Hyde is seated to Eoin McNeil's right.

Source: Courtesy of the Curran family.

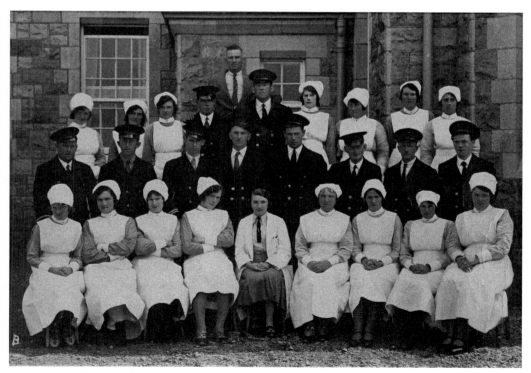

6. Staff at Ballinasloe District Asylum with English at the front centre (c.1917).

Source: Mattie Ganly. Used with permission.

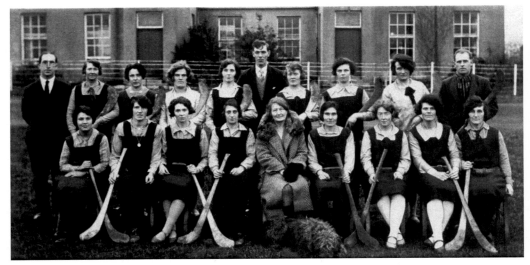

7. Ballinasloe Mental Hospital Camogie Team, 1928. Silver medalists in the 2nd Tailteann Games, Dublin, 1928.
Back Row: Dennis Coen, Kattie Manning, Annie Egan, Mary Shaughnessy, Delia Kilalea, Thomas Mulrenan, Peg Clarke, Katie Dolan, Mary Norton, Bill Burke. *Front Row:* Bridie Byrnes, Margaret Lyons, Mary Coghlan, Nell Mahon (captain), Dr Ada English, Mary E. Carroll, Winnie Clarke, Annie Finnerty, Nora King. Original photo by: Central Studios, 13 Nth. Earl St., Dublin.
Source: Ballinasloe Photo Gallery. Courtesy of Dr Damian Mac Con Uladh, Greece.

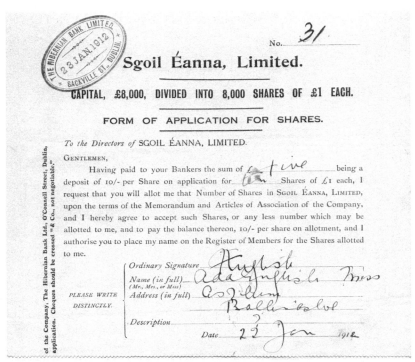

8. Share Certificate, signed by English. On 22 January 1912, English purchased shares in Patrick Pearse's school, Scoil Éanna Ltd., in an unsuccessful attempt to shore up the finance of the school. Within months, the company was in liquidation and investors only got 6d in the £ in respect of their donation.
Source: Courtesy of the Pearse Museum/OPW.

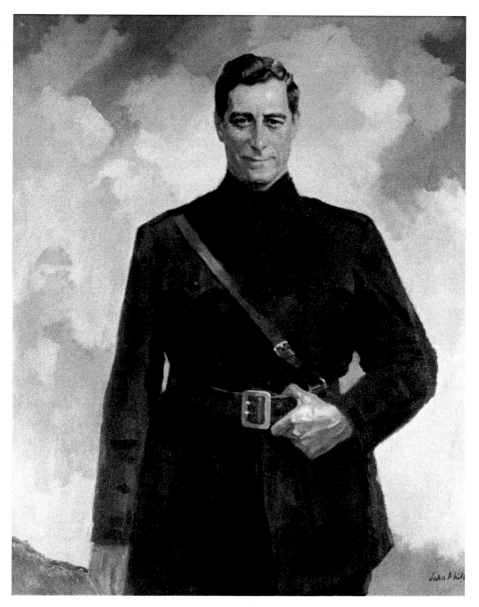

9. Cathal Brugha (1874-1922) by John F Kelly (Leinster House, Dublin). Brugha and English found common cause opposing the Anglo-Irish Treaty (1921) during the Civil War (1922-23).

Source: Image provided courtesy of the Houses of the Oireachtas.

The Asylum

Ḿ ENGLISH. Ada. ⌐ Ballinasloe, Co. Galway.

Age, about 45. (1921).

Professor.

Elected Sinn Fein M.P. for National University, Dublin, May 1921.

1st Medical Officer, Ballinasloe Lunatic Asylum, Co. Galway.

Present at a Sinn Fein Meeting in Galway Town on 1-1-18.

On 3-3-18 was reported to be President of the Local CUMANN-na-mBAN. which she organised.

Took a prominent part in the womens anti-conscription demonstration at Ballinasloe 9-6-18 and was the chief Organiser.

House searched 17-1-21. Various documents relating to Sinn Fein seized. and in consequence was

(? F.G.C.M.)

Arrested 19-1-21, and tried by D.C.M. at Galway 24-2-21. Sentenced to 9 months imprisonment without hard labour.

Released from Galway Prison 13-5-21 on grounds of ill-health and on giving an undertaking to reside outside Counties Galway and Mayo

Although not residing in Ballinasloe since her release, it is believed she has been active in connection with the Sinn Fein Movement.

Name appears in secret documents seized from Michael Collins as the Delegate from Co. Galway to the Annual Convention of Cumann-na-mBan 1919-1920.

ACTIVITIES SINCE THE TRUCE.

"Blood & Thunder"

After making a speech at Ballinasloe she proceeded openly to enlist members of the Cimann-na-mBan. (IX/0135).

Voted against Treaty on Sat 7.1.22.

Re-nominated as Anti-Treaty member for her present constituency to contest in elections June 1922.

Defeated at Poll for 3rd Dail.

Arrested by r.G. Troops, with four other members of Cumann na mBan, recently. ("Republican War News" No35, dated 10th -8-22)

---

10. Extract from War Office "Castle File No. 4168: Dr English, Ada" WO 35/206/75.

Source: Courtesy of The National Archives, Kew, Surrey, TW9 4DU UK.

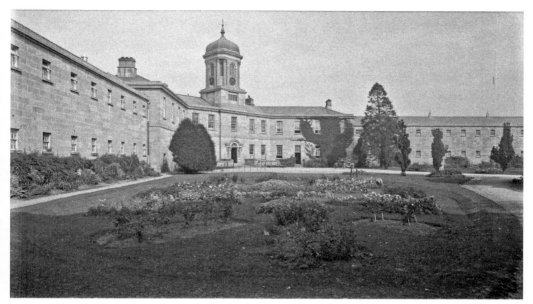

11. Asylum, Ballinasloe, Co Galway (1900-1920). English worked here for three decades, from 1904 onwards, finally becoming Resident Medical Superintendent in 1941.

Source: Eason Collection. Courtesy of the National Library of Ireland.

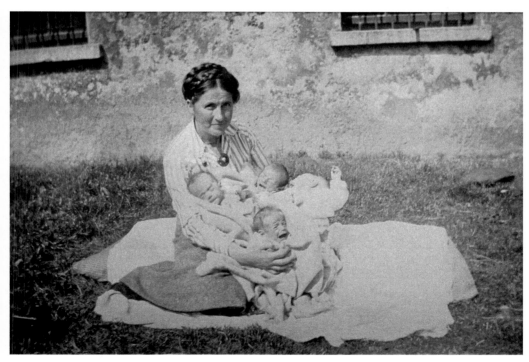

12. Dr Kathleen Lynn (1874-1955), co-founder of St Ultan's Hospital (1919) and Sinn Féin member of the Fourth Dáil (1923-27), who devoted her medical career to the care of infants and children, and the cause of public health.

Source: Reproduced by kind permission of the Royal College of Physicians of Ireland.

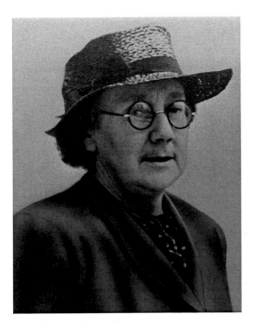

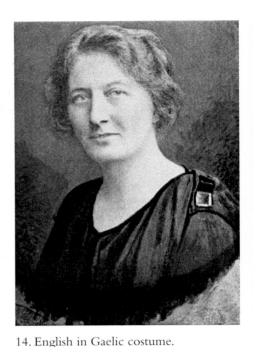

13. Dr Dorothy Price (1890–1954) served as a medical officer to a Cork brigade of the Irish Republican Army in the early 1920s, and went on to play a key role in the fight against tuberculosis in Ireland.

Source: Reproduced by kind permission of the Royal College of Physicians of Ireland.

14. English in Gaelic costume.

Source: Meenan, F.O.C., *Cecilia Street: The Catholic University School of Medicine, 1855-1931* (Dublin: Gill and Macmillan, 1987). Used with permission.

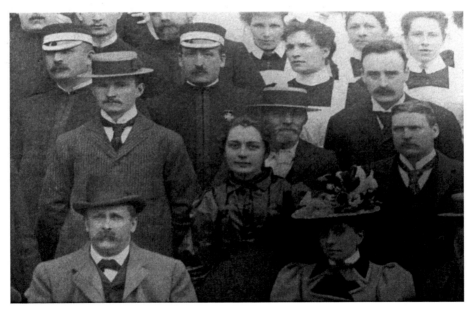

15. Dr Eleanora Fleury (1867-1960) (centre, without a hat c. 1897), worked in the Richmond and Portrane Asylums, Dublin and was arrested in 1923 for treating wounded republicans in Portrane. She spent three months in detention.

Source: St Brendan's Hospital Museum and Dr Aidan Collins.

1940 to 14 June 1940) but returned on the day of the Commissioner's first meeting.

The minutes of this meeting record receipt of a letter from the Department of Local Government and Public Health dated 11 June 1940, advising the Commissioner that the Minister was of the opinion that:

(1) Dr Lyons cannot be further trusted with the responsible duties of Resident Medical Superintendent. A reduction in rank should be considered forthwith.

(2) Suitable disciplinary action is necessary in the case of Dr Delaney … proposals in regard to Dr Delaney should be submitted as early as possible.

(3) The Matron should be retired on pension.

(4) Dr English, Assistant Medical Officer, in her evidence at the inquiry, took exception to a report made by the Resident Medical Superintendent to the Joint Committee to the effect that the Assistant Medical Officers did the minimum amount of work. She also felt aggrieved by a statement made by the Resident Medical Superintendent, at a meeting of the Committee, which reflected upon her veracity. The Resident Medical Superintendent agreed at the inquiry to express regret and withdraw the statement. The Minister is satisfied that Dr English has discharged her duties efficiently.

The Commissioner then 'declared the position of Resident Medical Superintendent vacant' and 'appointed Dr Adeline English [as] Acting Resident Medical Superintendent at £800 per annum without allowances except unfurnished house'. He 'promoted Dr B. Lyons [outgoing RMS] to the position of Medical Officer at Castlerea Branch Mental Asylum'; 'placed Dr J. Delaney on two years' probation with a reduction in his present salary of £100 per annum'; and 'asked the Matron to hand in her resignation and she agreed to tender her resignation that day'.[223] The minutes detailing these decisions were signed by 'Eithne Inglis, Acting RMS'.

The decisions were duly reported, without comment, in the *Irish Times*.[224] Reaction was more colourful at the July meeting of Roscommon County Council, the county in which Lyons's new place of work, Castlerea Branch Mental Asylum, was located. One Council member objected to the summary dissolution of the Committee in Ballinasloe:

Mrs Hannon said it was very ignominious the way they were turned out. She wished to make a protest against it and added that it was anything but nice the treatment that was given to Dr Lyons. They would never get a better man again. It was very badly done.[225]

Overall, the inquiry in Ballinasloe was an intensely interesting affair. It was revealing not only for the details that emerged regarding specific disputes, but also Lyons's evidence about the genuine difficulties he faced in running a large, complicated establishment such as Ballinasloe Mental Hospital. The hospital encompassed a vast campus, with buildings and farms, and large numbers of patients and staff. Lyons provided details of multiple problems between staff members which came to his attention, many of which were complicated, entrenched and apparently intractable.[226] Resolving these disputes in the institutional environment of a mental hospital was never going to be easy and Lyons's evidence to the inquiry demonstrated that the job of RMS was, in many ways, an impossible one.

The changes introduced following the inquiry were both sweeping and decisive, but were also complex. Matron O'Connor, for example, was 'retired on pension' following the inquiry,[227] but she remained a very popular figure in the mental hospital. In the month after the inquiry, she received special mention at the first meeting of the Commissioner Acting for the Dissolved Committee of Management:

> The matron, Mrs Harris O'Connor, is resigning after long, faithful and devoted service to the interests of the patients under her care, and of the whole Institution. The Staff desires to be associated in wishing her very many happy years in her well-earned leisure and to assure her of their regret and sorrow at her departure, and the patients will miss a kind and cheery friend who was always ready to listen sympathetically to their woes and do all she could to remedy them.[228]

These warm wishes were not unexpected: the much-valued Mrs O'Connor was not only a long-serving matron, but also daughter of Matt Harris, a nationalist and public representative in Ballinasloe, who died in 1890.[229] Harris had been a prominent figure in local and national affairs, and a friend of Charles Stewart Parnell, founder of the Irish Parliamentary Party; John Dillon, leader of the Irish Parliamentary Party; and Michael Davitt, founder of the Irish National Land League.

Resident Medical Superintendent English

By this time, as English again took over as acting RMS in 1940, the number of patients in the hospital had increased to 1887 (1,106 male, 781 female) and, of these, 461 were 'under treatment' (221 male, 195 female).[230] As with many such institutions in Ireland during this time, there were significant problems with the physical health of both patients and staff. In March 1941, for example, English, as acting RMS, reported that 'influenza has been widely spread through the house during the last month, particularly this last fortnight. Both patients and staff are affected…'[231]

Tuberculosis (TB) was also a substantial problem in Ballinasloe Mental Hospital at this time and the Inspector made particular reference to it following his inspection on 28 November 1939:

> One hundred and twenty-two patients died during the year, of this number 36 died of Pulmonary Tuberculosis, and six from General Tuberculosis. This is rather a high percentage of deaths from tuberculosis, and can scarcely be regarded as altogether unconnected with the overcrowded state of the institution.[232]

TB had been a long-standing problem in Irish mental hospitals[233] and was the single most common cause of death amongst inpatients toward the end of the 1800s.[234] In the early 1900s, when English arrived in Ballinasloe, TB accounted for over 25 per cent of deaths in Irish mental hospitals[235] and almost 16 per cent of all deaths in the Irish population.[236] Similar problems were reported in asylums in other countries.[237]

In 1907, Dr Conolly Norman, medical superintendent of the Richmond Asylum in Dublin,[238] drew the urgent attention of Richmond Asylum Joint Committee to the problem and recommended physical isolation of TB patients:

> I believe the desirability of isolation as far as possible in cases of pulmonary consumption will now be generally recognised… The present, therefore, seems to be a particularly suitable time to again draw attention to the great prevalence among our patients of tuberculosis consumption and the need that exists for some special provision for isolating sufferers from this disease. No large scheme of new construction or re-arrangement ought to be considered without a special view to this topic.[239]

Segregation remained an important element in the institutional management of TB for many decades and, in August 1933, 'Mr E. Boyd Barrett, architect … submitted plans of new buildings at Ballinasloe' to 'include TB hospital, admission hospital, chronic block, nurses' home, and doctor's residence'.[240] Works were duly performed and, in February 1940, the Committee of Management 'agreed that chronic patients would occupy the cream buildings, TB patients in the TB block, and new and recent admissions in the Admission Hospital'.[241] By July 1940, there were forty patients in the TB block.[242]

Other problems at Ballinasloe Mental Hospital during English's period as acting RMS related to the advent of World War II, for which many important (and not so important) precautions had to be taken: 'Owing to the danger of scarcity of tea, we have got a stock of cocoa', the Committee of Management heard.[243] More significantly, in July 1940, English reported to the Committee that 'the military have taken over the farm building block (since 27 June 1940), despite our protests to them, the Local Government Department and the Department of Defence… We are having trenches dug, air raid shelters provided and the military have been very kind and helpful to us in advice and supervision'.[244]

In June of the following year, English, who was once again acting RMS, was finally substantively 'appointed as resident medical superintendent of Ballinasloe and Castlerea Mental Hospitals'.[245] At this point, English was sixty-six years of age and had been working at Ballinasloe Mental Hospital for some thirty-seven years.

On becoming RMS, English continued the duties now familiar to her from her three decades working at the mental hospital. One of her duties was to inspect the various farmlands and buildings owned by the hospital. A patient drove her around in a horse and trap, with English carefully wrapped in a rug. On at least one occasion, the patient wrapped one of the assistant land steward's sons in a similar rug and drove him around on the pony and trap just to see patients and staff scramble to attention as they believed English had arrived.[246]

English occupied the post of RMS for fourteen months before, on 11 August 1942, she submitted her letter of resignation to the Committee of Management.[247] She retired from her post at University College Galway in 1943 and was succeeded by Cornelius McCarthy, also of Ballinasloe.[248] The following year, on 27 January 1944, English died at Mount Pleasant Nursing Home (later Portiuncula Hospital) in Ballinasloe.

Conclusion

English's obituary in the *East Galway Democrat* noted that she had been 'foremost in urging and helping the changes which transformed the then "Lunatic Asylum" to be one of the finest in the country' and 'developed occupational therapy to a high degree,' amongst other therapeutic innovations.[249] These were indeed notable achievements, but it is also true that, over her four decades in Ballinasloe, she had wrestled steadily and persistently with many of the less glamorous, apparently intractable day-to-day problems within the asylums, ranging from chronic overcrowding to industrial disputes, from tuberculosis and typhoid to an especially bitter dispute amongst staff, resulting in the Sworn Inquiry (1940) and English finally becoming RMS.

These kinds of problems were by no means unique to Ballinasloe. In 1924, in the midst of English's time in Ballinasloe, Edward Boyd Barrett SJ wrote an outspoken article about 'modern psycho-therapy and our asylums' in *Studies: An Irish Quarterly Review*:

> The rate of committals to asylums goes on increasing, and there exists no means of treating cases of incipient insanity. Curable nerve cases are allowed to develop into incurable cases. The public, ignorant and indifferent as regard mental disease, gives no encouragement to the setting up of nerve clinics or to the practice of the new methods of psycho-therapy.[250]

Boyd Barrett was especially concerned with the paucity of treatments provided and the unpleasant nature of the asylum environment:

> The most lamentable feature of the present asylum system is the absence of treatment. Apart from the many hardships that the unfortunate patients have to put up with − the poor and monotonous diet, the repulsive prison-like surroundings, the dreary exercise yards, the hideous clothing, the punishments for refectory patients, the uncongenial associates, the nerve-raking cries, the dirt and general gloom, the almost total absence of amusement and recreation − there is this appalling difference between the mental hospital (as an asylum should be) and the ordinary hospital, that in the latter each kind of disease is carefully treated by the best modern methods, whereas in the former no type of mental disease is fully treated.[251]

Twenty years later, in 1944, two years after English retired, an anonymous psychiatrist wrote a similarly outspoken article in *The Bell*, an Irish literary periodical:

> The history of insanity in this country does not differ from that in others. Its incidence was about the same; its causes were similar; the attitude of the public towards it was equally callous and the absence of any attempt at scientific treatment equally noticeable. In the early decades of the [nineteenth] century some differences became apparent. Neighbouring countries began to do something about it and their Governments took active steps in providing 'Asylums' for the mentally afflicted, but the Irish [*sic*] Government lagged behind and, even though many years have passed, that lag is still apparent.[252]

The anonymous psychiatrist stated that prior to the asylums of the 1800s the plight of the mentally ill was 'appalling', as they 'were regarded as outcasts' and 'chained down in the dark in filthy surroundings' or 'beaten and starved'.[253] The decades leading up to 1944, during English's career, had, however, seen significant improvement:

> The change has been a gradual one. First had to come the knowledge that insanity was not due to possession by evil spirits. It gradually oozed into the minds of the public that insanity was a disease. So, in time, the gaoler with the whip was replaced by the doctor. Then the old-fashioned doctor with his copious blood-letting and drastic medicinal treatment gave place, as generations passed, to the specialist; which brings us to the present time.[254]

As one such 'specialist', English played a key role in introducing such changes in Ballinasloe, one of Ireland's largest mental hospitals, over a period of almost four decades. The fact that English combined her professional work in the asylum with intensive political activity makes her contributions to both medicine and politics all the more remarkable.

Intriguingly, however, English was not alone in combining nationalist politics with progressive medical practice during this turbulent period in Ireland's history. The next chapter, Chapter Four, places English's life and career into the context of four other women doctors who were contemporaries of English and, like her, combined politics with medicine to very good effect.

Notes

1. E. Boyd Barrett, 'Modern psycho-therapy and our asylums', *Studies*, 13, 49 (March 1924), pp.9–43.
2. *East Galway Democrat*, 29 January 1944.
3. *Irish Press*, 28 January 1944.
4. A. O'Connor, 'Forget gender quotas, we need more Brigids in Dáil', *Irish Independent*, 12 May 2012.
5. M. Ó hÓgartaigh, '"Is there any need of you?" Women in medicine in Ireland and Australia', *Australian Journal of Irish Studies*, 4 (2004), pp.162–71.
6. Ó hÓgartaigh, *Kathleen Lynn*.
7. Ó hÓgartaigh, *Ireland in the 1930s*, pp.67–82; A. Mac Lellan, 'Dr Dorothy Price and the eradication of TB in Ireland', *Irish Medical News*, 19 May 2008.
8. B.D. Kelly, 'Mental health law in Ireland, 1821 to 1902: building the asylums', *Medico-Legal Journal*, 76, 1 (March 2008), pp.19–25; B.D. Kelly, 'Mental health law in Ireland, 1821 to 1902: dealing with the "increase of insanity in Ireland"', *Medico-Legal Journal*, 76, 1 (March 2008), pp.26–33.

9. M. Finnane, *Insanity and the Insane in Post-Famine Ireland* (London: Croom Helm, 1981), pp.18–47; B.D. Kelly, 'Mental illness in nineteenth-century Ireland: a qualitative study of workhouse records', *Irish Journal of Medical Science*, 173, 1 (January 2004), pp.53–5.

10. J. Robins, *Fools and Mad: A History of the Insane in Ireland* (Dublin: Institute of Public Administration, 1986).

11. Reynolds, *Grangegorman: Psychiatric Care in Dublin since 1815*; B.D. Kelly, 'One hundred years ago: the Richmond Asylum, Dublin in 1907', *Irish Journal of Psychological Medicine*, 24, 3 (September 2007), pp.108–14.

12. A. Williamson, 'The beginnings of state care for the mentally ill in Ireland', *Economic and Social Review (Ireland)*, 10, 1 (January 1970), pp.280–91.

13. D. Walsh and A. Daly, *Mental Illness in Ireland, 1750–2002: Reflections on the Rise and Fall of Institutional Care* (Dublin: Health Research Board, 2004).

14. L.D. Smith, 'The county asylum in the mixed economy of care, 1808–1845', in J. Melling and B. Forsythe (eds), *Insanity Institutions and Society, 1800–1914: A Social History of Madness in Comparative Perspective* (London and New York: Routledge, 1999), pp.33–47; L. Smith, *Lunatic Hospitals in Georgian England, 1750–1830 (Routledge Studies in the Social History of Medicine)* (London: Routledge, 2007).

15. A. Williamson, 'The beginnings of state care for the mentally ill in Ireland', pp.280–91.

16. O. Walsh, 'Gender and insanity in nineteenth-century Ireland', *Clio Medica/The Wellcome Series in the History of Medicine*, 73, 1 (January 2004), pp.69–93; B.D. Kelly, 'Mental health law in Ireland, 1821 to 1902: building the asylums', *Medico-Legal Journal*, 76, 1 (March 2008), pp.19–25.

17. A.-M. O'Neill, *Irish Mental Health Law* (Dublin: First Law Ltd, Dublin, 2005).

18. P. Prior, 'Dangerous lunacy: The misuse of mental health law in nineteenth-century Ireland', *Journal of Forensic Psychiatry and Psychology*, 14, 3 (December 2003), pp.525–41.

19. M. Reuber, 'The architecture of moral management: the Irish asylums (1801–1922)', *Psychological Medicine*, 26, 6 (November 1996), pp.1179–89; MacLoughlin, *Ballinasloe Inniú agus Inné*, p.76.

20. MacLoughlin, *Ballinasloe Inniú agus Inné*, p.76.

21. Walsh, O. 'A perfectly ordered establishment: Connaught District Lunatic Asylum (Ballinasloe)', in P.M. Prior (ed.), *Asylums, Mental Health Care and the Irish, 1800–2010* (Dublin: Irish Academic Press, 2011), pp.246–70.

22. *Irish Times*, 17 January 1885.

23. Inspectors of Lunatics, *The Forty-Second Report (With Appendices) of the Inspector of Lunatics (Ireland)* (Dublin: Thom and Co. for Her Majesty's Stationery Office, 1893).

24. Inspectors of Lunatics, *The Forty-Second Report (With Appendices) of the Inspector of Lunatics (Ireland)*, p.7.

25. MacLoughlin, *Ballinasloe Inniú agus Inné*, p.77.

26. D. Walsh, 'The ups and downs of schizophrenia in Ireland', *Irish Journal of Psychiatry*, 13, 2 (1992), pp.12–16; Walsh and Daly, *Mental Illness in Ireland, 1750–2002*; B.D. Kelly, 'Mental health law in Ireland, 1821 to 1902: dealing with the "increase of insanity in Ireland"', *Medico-Legal Journal*, 76, 1 (March 2008), pp.26–33.

27. O. Walsh, '"Tales from the big house": The Connacht District Lunatic Asylum in the late nineteenth century', *History Ireland*, 13, 6 (2005), pp.21–5.

28. *Medical Directory for 1905* (London: J. & A. Churchill, 1905), p.1414; *Irish Press*, 28 January 1944; *East Galway Democrat*, 29 January 1944; *Irish Times*, 29 January 1944; F. Clarke, 'English, Adeline ('Ada')', in J. McGuire and J. Quinn (eds), *Dictionary of Irish Biography: From the Earliest Times to the Year 2002 (Volume 3, D-F)* (Cambridge: Royal Irish Academy and Cambridge University Press, 2009), pp.626–7.

29. D. Healy, 'Irish psychiatry in the twentieth century', in H. Freeman and G.E. Berrios (eds), *150 Years of British Psychiatry. Volume II: The Aftermath* (London: Athlone Press, London, 1996), pp.268–91.

30. Minutes of the Proceedings of the Committee of Management of Ballinasloe District Asylum, 10 October 1904.

31. Ibid., 13 June 1904.

32. Ibid., 12 September 1904.

33. MacLoughlin, *Ballinasloe Inniú agus Inné*, pp.34–5.

34. *Connacht Tribune*, 21 March 1936.

35. *Irish Times*, 16 July 1904. See also: *Irish Times*, 8 July 1904.

36. *Irish Times*, 16 July 1904.

37. Ibid.

38. Kelly, *Between the Lines of History*, p.25.

39. D. Kelly, *Ballinasloe: From Garbally Park to the Fairgreen* (Dublin: Nonsuch, 2007), p.92; *Irish Press*, 28 January 1944; *East Galway Democrat*, 29 January 1944.

40. *Irish Press*, 28 January 1944; *East Galway Democrat*, 29 January 1944; F. Clarke, 'English, Adeline ('Ada')', in J. McGuire and J. Quinn (eds), *Dictionary of Irish Biography*, pp.626–7.

41. Kelly, *Between the Lines of History*, p.25.

42. J. Madden, *Fr John Fahy: Radical Republican and Agrarian Activist (1893–1969)* (Dublin: Columbia Press, 2012), pp.28–9.

43. MacLoughlin, *Ballinasloe Inniú agus Inné*, p.168.

44. Ibid., p.166.

45. D. Kelly, *Meadow of the Miracles: A History of the Diocese of Clonfert* (Strasbourg: Editions du Signe, 2006), p.73.

46. McNamara and Mooney, *Women in Parliament: 1918–2000*, p.79.

47. MacLoughlin, *Ballinasloe Inniú agus Inné*, p.168.

48. Minutes of the Proceedings of the Committee of Management of Ballinasloe District Asylum, 12 June 1916

49. Ibid., 11 July 1921.

50. *Connacht Tribune*, 21 March 1936.

51. Minutes of the Proceedings of the Committee of Management of Ballinasloe District Asylum, 14 February 1921.

52. C. Cox, *Negotiating Insanity in the Southeast of Ireland, 1820–1900* (Manchester and New York: Manchester University Press, 2012), p.17.

53. Reynolds, *Grangegorman: Psychiatric Care in Dublin since 1815*, pp.16–19.

54. B.D. Kelly, 'Dr William Saunders Hallaran and psychiatric practice in nineteenth-century Ireland', *Irish Journal of Medical Science*, 177, 1 (March 2008), pp.79–84.

55. W.S. Hallaran, *An Inquiry into the Causes producing the Extraordinary Addition to the Number of Insane together with Extended Observations on the Cure of Insanity with hints as to the Better Management of Public Asylums for Insane Persons* (Cork: Edwards and Savage, 1810), pp.46–7.

56. Hallaran, *An Inquiry into the Causes producing the Extraordinary Addition to the Number of Insane*, p.109.

57. J-É Esquirol. *Des Passions.* Paris: Didot Jeune, 1805.

58. E.T. Carlson and N. Dain, 'The psychotherapy that was moral treatment', *American Journal of Psychiatry*, 117 (December 1960), pp.519–24.

59. Robins, *Fools and Mad: A History of the Insane in Ireland*, pp.28–42.

60. E. Shorter, *A History of Psychiatry: From the Era of the Asylum to the Age of Prozac* (New York: John Wiley & Sons, 1997), pp.69–112.

61. W. Fogarty, *Dr Eamonn O'Sullivan: A Man Before His Time* (Dublin: Wolfhound Press, 2007).

62. E.N.M. O'Sullivan, *Textbook of Occupational Therapy: With Chief Reference to Psychological Medicine* (Oxford: Philosophical Library, 1955).

63. *East Galway Democrat*, 29 January 1944.

64. Minutes of the Proceedings of the Committee of Management of Ballinasloe District Asylum, 9 June 1942.

65. Anonymous, 'Irish Division', *Journal of Mental Science*, 63, 263 (1917), p.620.

66. B.D. Kelly, 'Physical sciences and psychological medicine: the legacy of Prof John Dunne', *Irish Journal of Psychological Medicine*, 22, 2 (2005), pp.67–72.

67. Anonymous, 'Irish Division', p.620.

68. Roscommon Herald, 13 February 1937 (reporting on the meeting of the Committee of Management of the Ballinasloe Mental Hospital which took place on 8 February 1937).

69. Minutes of the Proceedings of the Committee of Management of Ballinasloe District Asylum, 8 April 1940.

70. Anonymous. 'Ballinasloe Asylum', *Journal of Mental Science*, 62, 258 (1916), p.651.

71. MacLoughlin, *Ballinasloe Inniú agus Inné*, p.144; F. Clarke, 'English, Adeline ('Ada')', in J. McGuire and J. Quinn (eds), *Dictionary of Irish Biography*, pp.626–7.

72. Minutes of the Proceedings of the Committee of Management of Ballinasloe District Asylum, 12 August 1940. The hospital also had to pay a 'license' for the cinema, a situation which members of the Committee of Management described as a 'shame' and a 'disgrace' (*Connacht Tribune*, 15 June 1929; reporting on the meeting of the Committee of Management of the Ballinasloe Mental Hospital which took place on 10 June 1929).

73. Minutes of the Proceedings of the Committee of Management of Ballinasloe District Asylum, 9 September 1940.

74. Ibid., 14 October 1940.

75. MacLoughlin, *Ballinasloe Inniú agus Inné*, p.144.

76. S. Cherry and R. Munting, '"Exercise is the thing": Sport and the asylum c1850-1950', *International Journal of the History of Sport*, 22, 1 (January 2006), pp.42–58.

77. O. Walsh, 'Cure or Custody: Therapeutic Philosophy at the Connaught District Lunatic Asylum', in M.H. Preston and M. Ó hÓgartaigh (eds), *Gender and Medicine in Ireland, 1700–1950* (Syracuse, NY: Syracuse University Press, 2012), pp.69–85.

78. Hanniffy, Dr Liam, Assistant Inspector of Mental Hospitals (retired) and son of Mr John Hanniffy, assistant land steward, Mental Hospital, Ballinasloe, County Galway (interview in Portlaoise, County Laois, 27 May 2013).

79. *East Galway Democrat*, 13 June 1914.

80. S. Cherry and R. Munting, '"Exercise is the thing": Sport and the asylum c1850–1950', *International Journal of the History of Sport*, pp.42–58.

81. MacLoughlin, *Ballinasloe Inniú agus Inné*, pp.144–5.

82. *Irish Times*, 11 May 1907.

83. Minutes of the Proceedings of the Committee of Management of Ballinasloe District Asylum, 9 October 1916.

84. *Irish Times*, 14 October 1916.

85. *East Galway Democrat*, 29 January 1944; McNamara and Mooney, *Women in Parliament: 1918–2000*, p.79; F. Clarke, 'English, Adeline ('Ada')', in J. McGuire and J. Quinn (eds), *Dictionary of Irish Biography*, pp.626–7.

86. Minutes of the Proceedings of the Committee of Management of Ballinasloe District Asylum, 20 November 1939.

87. *East Galway Democrat*, 29 January 1944.

88. Shorter, *A History of Psychiatry*, pp.207–217.

89. T. Millon, *Masters of the Mind: Exploring the Story of Mental Illness from Ancient Times to the New Millennium* (Hoboken, NJ: John Wiley and Sons, 2004), pp.239–240.

90. E. Shorter and D. Healy, *Shock Therapy: A History of Electroconvulsive Treatment in Mental Illness* (New Brunswick, NJ and London: Rutgers University Press, 2007), p.23.

91. N. McCrae, 'A violent thunderstorm: Cardiazol treatment in British mental hospitals', *History of Psychiatry*, 17, 1 (March 2006), pp.67–90.

92. L.J.Von Meduna, Ladislas J.Von 'Versuche über die biologische Beeinflussung des Aflaubes der Schizophrenie', *Zeitschrift für die gesamte Neurologie und Psychiatrie*, 152, 1 (December 1935), pp.235–62.

93. N. McCrae, 'A violent thunderstorm: Cardiazol treatment in British mental hospitals', pp.67–90.

94. Reynolds, *Grangegorman: Psychiatric Care in Dublin since 1815*, p.264.

95. J. Dunne, 'Survey of modern physical methods of treatment for mental illness carried out in Grangegorman Mental Hospital', *Journal of the Medical Association of Eire*, 27, 157 (July 1950), pp.4–9; J. Dunne, 'The contribution of the physical sciences to psychological medicine', *Journal of Mental Science*, 102, 427 (April 1956), pp.209–20; B.D. Kelly, 'Physical sciences and psychological medicine: the legacy of Prof John Dunne', *Irish Journal of Psychological Medicine*, 22, 2 (July 2005), pp.67–72.

96. *East Galway Democrat*, 29 January 1944.

97. Minutes of the Proceedings of the Committee of Management of Ballinasloe District Asylum, 11 December 1939.

98. Reynolds, *Grangegorman: Psychiatric Care in Dublin since 1815*, p.264.

99. Dunne, 'Survey of modern physical methods of treatment for mental illness carried out in Grangegorman Mental Hospital', pp.4–9.

100. B.D. Kelly, 'Tuberculosis in the nineteenth-century asylum: Clinical cases from the Central Criminal Lunatic Asylum, Dundrum, Dublin', in P.M. Prior (ed.), *Asylums, Mental Health Care and the Irish, 1800–2010*, pp.205–20.

101. *Irish Times*, 31 May 1913.

102. *Connacht Tribune*, 18 March 1933.

103. *Connacht Tribune*, 13 January 1940.

104. Sworn Inquiry: Death of Patient by Drowning (L2/102) (318/27) (22017/1939) HLTH/SL2/98 (National Archives, Bishop Street, Dublin, Ireland).

105. Ibid.

106. Ibid.

107. Ibid.

108. Sworn Inquiry: Death of Patient (L2/102) (1927) HLTH/SL2/98 (National Archives, Bishop Street, Dublin, Ireland).

109. F. Clarke, 'English, Adeline ('Ada')', in J. McGuire and J. Quinn (eds), *Dictionary of Irish Biography*, pp.626–7.

110. M. Clancy, 'On the "Western Outpost": Local government and women's suffrage in county Galway', in G. Moran (ed.), *Galway: History and Society – Interdisciplinary Essays on the History of an Irish County* (Dublin: Geography Publications, 1996), pp.557–87.

111. *Irish Press*, 28 January 1944; *East Galway Democrat*, 29 January 1944; McNamara and Mooney, *Women in Parliament: 1918–2000*, p.79.

112. Finnerty, Mr Peter, Kiltormer, County Galway (interview in Ballinasloe, Country Galway on 3 May 2013).

113. 'Blessings be with you' (in Irish).

114. MacLoughlin, *Ballinasloe Inniú agus Inné*, p.77.

115. Madden, *Fr John Fahy*, pp.28–9.

116. *East Galway Democrat*, 19 January 1929 (reporting on the meeting of the Committee of Management of the Ballinasloe Mental Hospital, 14 January 1929).

117. MacLoughlin, *Ballinasloe Inniú agus Inné*, p.77.

118. Our Correspondent, 'Ballinasloe Lunatic Asylum', *Journal of Mental Science*, 62, 257 (1916), p.467.

119. *Connacht Tribune*, 15 June 1929 (reporting on the meeting of the Committee of Management of the Ballinasloe Mental Hospital, 10 June 1929).

120. *Roscommon Champion*, 11 November 1935 (reporting on the meeting of the Committee of Management of the Ballinasloe Mental Hospital, 6 November 1935); *Irish Independent*, 18 December 1937 (reporting on the meeting of the Committee of Management of the Ballinasloe Mental Hospital, 13 December 1937).

121. *Connacht Tribune*, 13 March 1937.

122. B.D. Kelly, 'One hundred years ago: the Richmond Asylum, Dublin in 1907', *Irish Journal of Psychological Medicine*, 24, 3 (2007), pp.108–14.

123. *Irish Times*, 21 November 1928. For more on the emergence of the insanity defence in Ireland, see: F. McAuley, *Insanity, Psychiatry and Criminal Responsibility* (Dublin: Round Hall Press, 1993); B.D. Kelly, 'Criminal insanity in nineteenth-century Ireland, Europe and the United States: cases, contexts and controversies', *International Journal of Law and Psychiatry*, 32, 6 (2009), pp.362–8.

124. *Connacht Tribune*, 15 June 1929 (reporting on the meeting of the Committee of Management of the Ballinasloe Mental Hospital, 10 June 1929).

125. *East Galway Democrat*, 19 January 1929 (reporting on the meeting of the Committee of Management of the Ballinasloe Mental Hospital, 14 January 1929).

126. *East Galway Democrat*, 18 January 1930 (reporting on the meeting of the Committee of Management of the Ballinasloe Mental Hospital, 13 January 1930).
127. Minutes of the Committee of Management of the Ballinasloe Mental Hospital, 11 November 1929.
128. *East Galway Democrat*, 16 November 1929.
129. A. McCabe and C. Mulholland, 'The red flag over the asylum: The Monaghan Asylum soviet of 1919', in P.M. Prior (ed.), *Asylums, Mental Health Care and the Irish, 1800–2010*, pp.23–43.
130. A.J. Sheridan, 'The impact of political transition on psychiatric nursing – a case study of twentieth-century Ireland', *Nursing Inquiry*, 13, 4 (2006), pp.289–299.
131. *Irish Times*, 16 July 1923.
132. *Irish Times*, 10 September 1924. See also: *Irish Times*, 16 February 1926.
133. *Irish Times*, 16 September 1924.
134. *The Times*, 10 September 1924. For further reports, see: *Nottingham Evening Post*, 9 September 1924; *Derby Daily Telegraph*, 9 September 1924; *Gloucester Citizen*, 9 September 1924; *Hull Daily Mail*, 9 September 1924; *Derby Daily Telegraph*, 10 September 1924.
135. *Irish Times*, 10 September 1924.
136. Some of these disputes were played out in the courts; e.g. *Irish Independent*, 22 June 1930, 23 January 1930 and 25 January 1930. These issues were also continually discussed at meetings of the Committee of Management of the Ballinasloe Mental Hospital (e.g. *Connacht Tribune*, 18 July 1931 (reporting on the meeting of the Committee of Management of the Ballinasloe Mental Hospital, 13 July 1931)).
137. *Irish Times*, 8 October 1938.
138. *Roscommon Champion*, 11 November 1935 (reporting on the meeting of the Committee of Management of the Ballinasloe Mental Hospital, 6 November 1935).
139. Ibid.
140. *Connacht Tribune*, 21 March 1936.
141. Ibid.
142. *Roscommon Herald*, 14 November 1936 (reporting on the meeting of the Committee of Management of the Ballinasloe Mental Hospital, 9 November 1936).
143. Minutes of the Proceedings of the Committee of Management of the Ballinasloe Mental Hospital, 9 November 1936.
144. *Irish Times*, 1 December 1936.
145. *Irish Times*, 12 December 1936.
146. Ibid.
147. *Irish Times*, 22 January 1929.
148. *Roscommon Herald*, 13 February 1937 (reporting on the meeting of the Committee of Management of the Ballinasloe Mental Hospital, 8 February 1937).
149. Ibid.
150. *Official Report of Dáil Éireann*, 3 February 1937.
151. Ibid.
152. Ibid.
153. *Roscommon Herald*, 13 February 1937 (reporting on the meeting of the Committee of Management of the Ballinasloe Mental Hospital, 8 February 1937).

154. Hanniffy, Dr Liam, Assistant Inspector of Mental Hospitals (retired) and son of Mr John Hanniffy,assistant land steward, Mental Hospital, Ballinasloe, County Galway (interview in Portlaoise, County Laois, 27 May 2013).

155. *Connacht Tribune*, 13 March 1937 (reporting on the meeting of the Committee of Management of the Ballinasloe Mental Hospital, 8 March 1937).

156. Ibid.

157. *Roscommon Herald*, 15 May 1937 (reporting on the meeting of the Committee of Management of the Ballinasloe Mental Hospital, 10 May 1937).

158. *Roscommon Herald*, 17 July 1937 (reporting on the meeting of the Committee of Management of the Ballinasloe Mental Hospital, 12 July 1937).

159. Minutes of the Proceedings of the Committee of Management of Ballinasloe District Asylum, 10 July 1939.

160. Minutes of the Proceedings of the Committee of Management of Ballinasloe District Asylum, 14 August 1939.

161. *Irish Times*, 11 July 1939; See also: *Irish Independent*, 6 January 1940.

162. During the ensuing inquiry, the chairman stated that 'Fr Hughes is exonerated, and cleared already' (Sworn Inquiry: Request by Committee for Sworn Inquiry Re Management of Institution since 1934: Unfavourable Press Reports re Administration etc., Lack of Harmony between Officers of Institution (L2/102) (1940) HLTH/SL2/98 (National Archives, Bishop Street, Dublin, Ireland) (hereafter referred to 'Inquiry'), p.131).

163. Cox, *Negotiating Insanity in the Southeast of Ireland, 1820–1900*, p.92.

164. *Irish Times*, 11 July 1939.

165. Ibid.

166. *Irish Times*, 26 August 1939.

167. Minutes of the Proceedings of the Committee of Management of Ballinasloe District Asylum, 8 January 1940.

168. Inquiry, cover sheet.

169. *Irish Times*, 4 January 1940.

170. *Irish Times*, 4 January 1940; *Irish Independent*, 6 January 1940.

171. Inquiry, p.2.

172. Inquiry, pp.2–3.

173. Inquiry, p.5.

174. Ibid.

175. Ibid.

176. Ibid.

177. Ibid., p.5–6.

178. Ibid., p.8.

179. Ibid., pp.9, 13.

180. Ibid., p.10.

181. Ibid.

182. Ibid., p.12.

183. Ibid., p.25.

184. Ibid., p.22.

185. Ibid.

186. Ibid.

187. Ibid.
188. Ibid. See also: *Irish Independent*, 6 January 1940.
189. Inquiry, p.23.
190. Ibid., p.25.
191. Ibid.
192. Inquiry, p.27. See also: *Irish Independent*, 6 January 1940.
193. Inquiry, pp.24, 29.
194. *Irish Times*, 26 August 1939.
195. Inquiry, p.30.
196. Inquiry, p.24.
197. Inquiry, pp.37–63, 89–90, pp.105–8.
198. Inquiry, pp.68, 91–2, 120.
199. *Irish Times*, 6 January 1940.
200. Inquiry, p.109.
201. Inquiry, p.110.
202. Inquiry, p.87.
203. Ibid.
204. Ibid.
205. Inquiry, pp.111, 121–4, 142–3. Some of Lyons's concerns about specific members of nursing staff were explored in some depth at the meeting of the Committee of Management of the Ballinasloe Mental Hospital on 9 August 1937 (see *East Galway Democrat*, 14 August 1937); significant difficulties in relation to the steward were discussed by Lyons and others at the Committee meeting of 13 September 1937 (see *Irish Independent*, 18 September 1937); and Lyons's further concerns about nursing and medical staff were discussed at the Committee meeting of 13 November 1937 (see *East Galway Democrat*, 18 November 1937).
206. *Irish Times*, 5 January 1940.
207. Inquiry, p.127.
208. Inquiry, p.133.
209. Inquiry, p.126.
210. Inquiry, p.140.
211. Inquiry, p.88.
212. Inquiry, p.98.
213. Inquiry, p.100.
214. Inquiry, p.101.
215. Inquiry, p.100.
216. Inquiry, p.101.
217. Inquiry, p.100.
218. Inquiry, p.101. See also: *Irish Press*, 5 January 1940.
219. Inquiry, p.126.
220. *Connacht Sentinel*, 16 March 1940.
221. Minutes of the Meeting of the Commissioner Administering the Affairs of the Ballinasloe Mental Hospital, 14 June 1940.
222. Ibid.
223. Ibid.
224. *Irish Times*, 22 June 1940.

225. *East Galway Democrat*, 13 July 1940.

226. In addition to the disputes already detailed, there were disputes between medical and nursing staff.

227. Minutes of the Meeting of the Commissioner Administering the Affairs of the Ballinasloe Mental Hospital, 14 June 1940.

228. Minutes of Proceedings of the Commissioner Acting for the Dissolved Committee of Management of Ballinasloe Mental Hospital, 8 July 1940.

229. MacLoughlin, *Ballinasloe Inniú agus Inné*, pp.163–4.

230. Minutes of the Proceedings of the Committee of Management of Ballinasloe District Asylum, 14 August 1939.

231. Ibid., 11 March 1941.

232. Ibid., 8 April 1940.

233. B.D. Kelly, 'Tuberculosis in the nineteenth-century asylum: Clinical cases from the Central Criminal Lunatic Asylum, Dundrum, Dublin', in P.M. Prior (ed.), *Asylums, Mental Health Care and the Irish, 1800–2010* (Dublin: Irish Academic Press, 2011), pp.205–20.

234. Inspectors of Lunatics (Ireland). *The Forty-Second Report (With Appendices) of the Inspectors of Lunatics (Ireland) 1892* (Dublin: Alexander Thom and Company (Limited) for Her Majesty's Stationery Office, 1893), p.7.

235. Finnane, *Insanity and the Insane in Post-Famine Ireland*, p.137.

236. G. Jones, 'The Campaign Against Tuberculosis in Ireland, 1899–1914', in E. Malcolm and G. Jones (eds), *Medicine, Disease and the State in Ireland, 1650–1940* (Cork: Cork University Press, 1999), pp.158–76.

237. P. McCandless, 'Curative asylum, custodial hospital: the South Carolina Lunatic Asylum and State Hospital, 1828-1920', in R. Porter and D. Wright (eds), *The Confinement of the Insane: International Perspectives, 1800–1965* (Cambridge: Cambridge University Press, 2003), pp.173–92.

238. Reynolds, *Grangegorman: Psychiatric Care in Dublin since 1815*; B.D. Kelly, 'One hundred years ago: the Richmond Asylum, Dublin in 1907', *Irish Journal of Psychological Medicine*, 24, 3 (2007), pp.108–14.

239. J. Conolly Norman, *Richmond Asylum Joint Committee Minutes* (Dublin: Richmond Asylum, 1907), p.540.

240. *Irish Independent*, 19 August 1933 (reporting on the meeting of the Committee of Management of the Ballinasloe Mental Hospital, 14 August 1933).

241. Minutes of the Proceedings of the Committee of Management of Ballinasloe District Asylum, 12 February 1940.

242. Ibid., 8 July 1940. See also: *East Galway Democrat*, 13 July 1940.

243. Minutes of the Proceedings of the Committee of Management of Ballinasloe District Asylum, 14 January 1940.

244. Ibid., 8 July 1940. See also: *East Galway Democrat*, 13 July 1940.

245. Ibid., 10 June 1941.

246. Hanniffy, Dr Liam, Assistant Inspector of Mental Hospitals (retired) and son of Mr John Hanniffy, assistant land steward, Mental Hospital, Ballinasloe, County Galway (interview in Portlaoise, County Laois, 27 May 2013).

247. Minutes of the Proceedings of the Committee of Management of Ballinasloe District Asylum, 11 August 1942.

248. Murray, *Galway: A Medico-Social History*, p.200; F. Clarke, 'English, Adeline ('Ada')', in J. McGuire and J. Quinn (eds), *Dictionary of Irish Biography*, pp.626–7.
249. *East Galway Democrat*, 29 January 1944.
250. E. Boyd Barrett, 'Modern psycho-therapy and our asylums', *Studies*, 13, 49 (March 1924), pp.9–43.
251. Boyd Barrett, 'Modern psycho-therapy and our asylums', p.30.
252. Psychiatrist, 'Insanity in Ireland', *The Bell*, 7, 4 (January 1944), pp.303–4.
253. Psychiatrist, 'Insanity in Ireland', p.304.
254. Ibid., p.305.

CHAPTER FOUR

———— ℘ ℭ ————

Revolution: Women Doctors in Early Twentieth-Century Ireland, 1900–42

E nglish practiced medicine during a period of uniquely intense social and political change in Ireland, throughout which there were significant problems with the establishment and maintenance of effective public health services.[1] English belonged to a remarkable group of Irish women doctors, each of whom made substantial contributions to the development of Irish medical services and improvement of social conditions, especially for children, the poor, the socially excluded and the mentally ill. These figures include Dr Kathleen Lynn, Dr Dorothy Price, Dr Brigid Lyons Thornton and Dr Eleonora Fleury. This chapter examines each of these figures in turn and compares their lives and careers with those of English.

Dr Kathleen Lynn (1874–1955)

There are particular parallels between the life and career of English and those of Dr Kathleen Lynn. Lynn was born in Mullaghfarry, near Killala in County Mayo.[2] Like English, Lynn grew up during a period of intense political activity, especially in Mayo where, in October 1879, the Irish National Land League was founded, with the aim of supporting tenant farmers in their conflicts with landlords regarding rent and land ownership.

Like English, Lynn was born into a relatively affluent family: Lynn's father was a Church of Ireland clergyman who, in 1882, was appointed to the estate of the Guinness family in Cong, County Mayo. Despite this relatively privileged childhood, Lynn, like English, was familiar with the difficulties of the time and, recognising that people saw their local doctor as a source of hope, decided to study medicine.[3]

Lynn received her initial schooling from a governess in Cong and enjoyed further education in Manchester and Dusseldorf. She received secondary schooling at Alexandra College in Dublin and, like English, attended the Catholic University School of Medicine in Dublin, where she enrolled in 1894. Despite her Church of Ireland background, Lynn could not attend the University of Dublin (Trinity College) because it did not admit women until 1904 and even then there were limitations: up until 1930, women under the age of eighteen years were barred from the study of anatomy and physiology at Trinity.[4]

Lynn quickly distinguished herself during her medical studies: she came first in practical anatomy in 1896; won the Barker Anatomical Prize in 1898; and won the Hudson Prize and silver medal on graduating in June 1899,[5] four years before English.[6] After graduation, Lynn was refused a position as a resident doctor at the Adelaide Hospital but gained experience at the Rotunda Hospital, the Royal Victoria Eye and Ear Hospital, and Sir Patrick Dun's Hospital in Dublin. Lynn completed postgraduate study in the United States and was awarded fellowship of the Royal College of Surgeons in 1909, the third woman so honoured.[7]

By this time, Lynn was deeply involved with the women's suffrage movement, having become a member of the executive committee of the Irish Women's Suffrage and Local Government Association in 1903.[8] In 1912, she attended suffragette hunger-strikers as medical officer.[9] Like English, Lynn was also deeply involved in Irish republican politics and, specifically, Cumann na mBan.[10] In Lynn's own words: 'I was converted to republicanism through suffrage. I saw that people got the wrong impression about suffrage and that led me to examine the Irish question.'[11]

At the invitation of James Connolly, Lynn gave first-aid lessons to members of the Irish Citizen Army (ICA, founded in 1913) and later became chief medical officer and a captain with the organisation.[12] This involvement parallels English's work as a medical officer with the Irish Volunteers (Óglaigh na hÉireann), also founded in 1913, with similar aims.[13]

During the Dublin Lock Out, a major industrial dispute involving tens of thousands of Dublin workers, Lynn worked in the soup kitchens, alongside her friend, fellow nationalist and distant cousin,[14] Constance Markievicz. Two years later, consistent with her prominence in the ICA, Lynn was actively involved in the 1916 Easter Rising in Dublin. In the weeks leading up to the Rising, Lynn assisted Connolly and Willie Pearse with logistics and preparations for military activity, and stored ammunition from Belfast in her home on Belgrave Road in Rathmines.[15]

The night before the Rising, Connolly ordered Lynn to spend the night at the house of Jennie Wyse Power, so that Lynn would be rested for the difficult days ahead.[16] During the Rising itself, Lynn took care of the sick and injured in Dublin's city centre[17] and served at the centre of action in Dublin's City Hall.[18] There, she tended to the wounded, including the first fatality amongst the rebels, Captain Sean Connolly.[19] In due course, Lynn, as highest ranking officer, tendered the republican surrender at City Hall[20] and when asked about her precise role responded that she was 'a Red Cross doctor and a belligerent'.[21]

English, too, had connections with the 1916 Rising, reportedly serving as medical officer with the Irish Volunteers in County Galway, led by Liam Mellows who was, like Lynn, a friend of both Connolly and Markievicz.[22] Both Connolly and Pearse were to die as a result of the Rising. Lynn was imprisoned in Ship Street Barracks in Dublin for a week, where she promptly instigated a de-lousing regime,[23] before being transferred to Kilmainham Gaol[24] and then deported to Coltsford, near Bath in England.[25]

By the end of August 1916 Lynn was back in Dublin[26] and, in 1917, she became a member of the executive of Sinn Féin.[27] Lynn's concern with health had a strong influence on her involvement with Sinn Féin: in February 1918 she co-authored the first public health charter, and in April 1919 she submitted a report on the influenza pandemic to the Sinn Féin Árd Fheis.[28] Lynn was deeply concerned about venereal disease and in February 1918 addressed the matter in a health circular co-written with Thomas Hynes, Sinn Féin's other co-director of health.[29]

English, too, was a member of Sinn Féin, and, in 1921, one of six party women elected to the Second Dáil, which supported the truce in the War of Independence.[30] Both English and Lynn opposed the Anglo–Irish Treaty, signed on 6 December 1921. During the subsequent Civil War, Lynn was based in Tipperary and Waterford, where her medical skills were extremely valuable for the anti-Treaty side.[31]

In 1921 Lynn was elected to the Sinn Féin Árd Comhairle standing committee and became one of the four vice-presidents of the party.[32] In 1923 she was elected as a Sinn Féin member of the Fourth Dáil,[33] just as English had been to the Second Dáil two years earlier. Lynn, however, did not take up her seat, in line with all anti-Treaty republicans at the time. Lynn was defeated in the 1927 general election, an outcome she faced philosophically: 'God knows best.'[34]

Lynn remained politically active for many more years after this, having been elected to Rathmines and Rathgar Urban District Council in 1920[35] and serving there for ten years.[36] Other members of the Council included Lynn's long-time friend, Madeleine ffrench-Mullen, and Hanna Sheehy Skeffington, a nationalist suffragette and co-founder of the Irish Women's Franchise League in 1908. Lynn also remained faithful to Cumann na mBan, long after many other members drifted away, often to join Fianna Fáil.[37]

Like English, Lynn was connected with 'Miss MacSwiney's Dáil' which met at the Rotunda in Dublin on 22 January 1929.[38] It was the view of Mary MacSwiney and her supporters that the new Dáil, formed after the Civil War, did not represent a legitimate government for Ireland, and she established 'Miss MacSwiney's Dáil' as an alternative, *real* government for the country. MacSwiney's group of 'legislators' in January 1929 comprised various republicans and anti-Treaty activists including the irrepressible Lynn. English was listed as an 'absentee member', not present on the day but clearly supportive of the cause.[39]

Like English, Lynn combined her political involvements with pioneering medical work. Sometimes the worlds of politics and medicine collided: in 1918, Lynn was arrested and imprisoned in Arbour Hill Prison, only to have the hospitals committee of Dublin Corporation petition for her release. To secure release, Lynn agreed to sign an undertaking: 'I Kathleen Lynn undertake on my honour if released from custody to take no part in politics, and not to leave the area of the Dublin Metropolitan Police.' Once released, however, she made her way to the Sinn Féin Árd Fheis in her capacity as director of health.[40]

Whereas English devoted her working life to the mentally ill, Lynn worked tirelessly to promote the health of children, and, especially, reduce infant mortality: in 1919, some 164 of every 1,000 infants born in Dublin died from preventable diseases.[41] Against this background, Lynn and ffrench-Mullen, in May 1919, established St Ultan's Hospital for Infants in Dublin with the aim of treating and supporting infants and mothers, and reducing infant mortality.[42]

Just as English's nationalist outlook was apparent in the Ballinasloe Asylum, so too was Lynn's politicised outlook apparent at St Ultan's: many hospital activities were advertised in Irish; many members of staff and supporters shared Lynn's nationalist views; and Lynn clearly saw her hospital work as contributing to Irish national regeneration.[43] To this end, St Ultan's was a truly pioneering institution and developed one of the first 'Montessori wards' in the world, while Lynn maintained a correspondence with Maria Montessori, the physician and philosopher of education, who visited St Ultan's in 1934.[44]

The 1930s saw the emergence of very significant political difficulties with the development of hospital care for children in Ireland, in which Lynn was deeply involved. In particular, the proposed amalgamation of St Ultan's with the National Children's Hospital on Harcourt Street generated significant conflict between Lynn and the Roman Catholic Archbishops Drs Byrne and McQuaid.[45] The dispute involved politics, religion and, tragically, health. Ultimately, Lynn could not prevail over the power of the Catholic Church and her relationship with the official Church suffered significantly as a result.

Lynn remained, however, highly active in medicine throughout the 1940s. In 1949 the National BCG Centre was established at St Ultan's Hospital and Lynn, like English[46] and many others, devoted considerable time and thought to the broader problems presented by TB. Lynn died on 14 September 1955 and was buried in the family plot in Deansgrange cemetery in Dublin with full military honours.[47]

Shortly after her death, the *Irish Times* published an 'appreciation' of Lynn, noting that 'by the death of Dr Kathleen Lynn Ireland has lost one of the most remarkable women of this century'.[48] Lynn's political and medical activities were detailed, and Lynn's life-long dedication to the care of infants was highlighted:

> In April 1955 Dr Lynn attended her out-patients' department for the last time. She was tired, old, and very ill. She had seen hundreds of thousands of babies in the 36 years since the hospital was founded. A mother came in with her first baby. The mother told me afterwards that 'Dr Lynn turned, smiled at me and looked at my baby as if it were the only baby in the world.' This is a tribute which very few of us can hope to earn.[49]

The similarities between Lynn and English are substantial, although not complete. Both women had relatively privileged childhoods but were also exposed to the suffering of others as children; both were amongst the first generation of female medical graduates in Ireland; both devoted their lives to pioneering medical work; both held strong nationalist views; both were connected with the War of Independence and Civil War; both spent periods of time in custody as a result of their political activities; and both entered the official political process – English as a Sinn Féin member of the Second Dáil and Lynn as a Sinn Féin member of the Fourth Dáil.

In addition, both Lynn and English were strong supporters of women's rights – English consistently opposed male chauvinism[50] and Lynn was deeply involved with the women's suffrage movement[51] – and, in 1917, pro-actively sought out significant positions for women in the reformed Sinn Féin.[52] Lynn also, in September 1917, co-wrote (with ffrench-Mullen) and distributed 25,000 copies of a pamphlet urging women to assert their political rights, funding their project by holding a raffle for a republican flag.[53]

Despite these similarities, there are also significant differences between the lives of Lynn and English. Lynn came from a strong Church of Ireland family, whereas English was Roman Catholic. Lynn devoted her life to the care of children, whereas English chose to work with the mentally ill. While neither woman married or had children, Lynn enjoyed the long-term companionship of ffrench-Mullen.[54] In addition, while Lynn left behind a detailed diary documenting her personal, medical and political activities, English did not leave any known personal account of her life. This makes it significantly challenging, although not impossible, to obtain a granular understanding of the thoughts, opinions and motivations that underpinned English's life and work.

Overall, it is apparent that there are remarkable similarities between the lives and careers of Lynn and English in terms of their medical careers, political activities and, to a certain extent, personal lives. Moreover, the lives of both women demonstrate significant similarities with those of three other women doctors who were, to greater or lesser degrees, their contemporaries: Dr Dorothy Price, Dr Brigid Lyons Thornton and Dr Eleonora Fleury. Price is considered next.

Dr Dorothy Price (1890–1954)

Like English and Lynn, Dr Dorothy Price combined progressive medical practice with nationalist political activism. Price was born Dorothy Stopford in Dublin in 1890. Her father, Jemmett Stopford, was a well-to-do Protestant accountant[55] and her maternal grandfather, Evory Kennedy, was master of the Rotunda Lying-In Hospital. Price's aunt was Alice Stopford-Green,[56] a celebrated historian who played an important role in cultural nationalism in Ireland in the early 1900s, along with artists such as Beatrice Elvery, Lily Yeats and Elizabeth Yeats, and writers such as Lady Gregory, the celebrated dramatist and folklorist.[57] Alice Stopford Green also spoke at nationalist public meetings, assisted financially with procuring arms, trained in first aid and co-founded a committee to campaign against conscription in 1918.[58] With this family background, it is unsurprising that Price herself developed strong nationalist views, despite her Protestant upbringing.

Like Lynn, Price received her early education from a governess in Dublin. When Price's father died from typhoid fever in 1902, the family moved to London where Price attended the progressive St Paul's Girls School as a foundation scholarship student.[59] After school, Price spent time working with the Charitable Organisation Society and displayed a keen interest in social work.

In 1916, Price returned to Ireland and enrolled to study medicine in Trinity College, Dublin.[60] Despite her clear academic ability and dedication to medicine, the Dublin University Biological Association refused Price entry to the Association because she was a woman.[61] The Association did not admit women as full members until 1941.

Price qualified as a doctor in 1921 and, after failing to secure employment in Dublin, went to work in Kilbrittain Dispensary in west Cork.[62] Here, Price encountered her first cases of TB, an illness which formed the focus of much of her subsequent work in medicine. Price was especially moved by the deaths of mothers and infants from TB, and lamented the state of medical knowledge and research into the topic in Ireland.[63] In Kilbrittain, Price also witnessed an outbreak of diphtheria resulting from poor hygiene which, she felt, could be addressed through simple reforms in conditions at the village.[64]

During her time in Kilbrittain, Price's political views evolved significantly and she served as medical officer to a Cork brigade of the Irish Republican Army (IRA), and later proudly sported a gold watch given to her by the IRA. Price's short history of the IRA in Cork clearly demonstrates her deep knowledge of its operations in the area.[65] In Kilbrittain, Price also received instructions from Cumann na mBan to lecture on first aid to the local branch of the organisation.[66] These activities are very similar to those of English, who, like Price, had early involvement with various nationalist groups as a medical officer and organized Red Cross lectures in Ballinasloe during the two World Wars.[67]

Price worked in Kilbrittain from 1921 to 1923, and then became a consultant physician at St Ultan's Infant Hospital in Dublin (co-founded by Lynn), consultant to the Royal National Hospital for Consumption in Ireland and the Sunshine Home (Stillorgan), and clinical assistant for children at the Royal City of Dublin Hospital.[68] In 1925, she married District Justice W.G. Price.

Price travelled extensively to observe medical practice in Italy, Sweden, Denmark and Germany. She taught herself German in order to read German-language text books, and corresponded with experts on the subject of TB, including Dr Walter Pagel in England and Professor Arvid Wallgren in Sweden.[69] In Vienna, Price went on ward rounds with Professor Hamburger, an expert on the use of tuberculin to diagnose TB. This was to prove a uniquely formative experience for Price.

On returning to Ireland, Price was dismayed to find that her new ideas from the continent were generally dismissed by colleagues, who traditionally looked to England rather than the continent for medical innovations. This was regrettable: TB was a major public health problem in Ireland and contemporary treatments were sharply limited in their scope and effectiveness.

During the second decade of the twentieth century, however, the Bacillus Calmette–Guérin (BCG) vaccination was developed by Léon Charles Albert Calmette and Jean-Marie Camille Guérin at the Institut Pasteur de Lille in

France. The vaccination, intended to protect recipients from TB, was first used in humans in 1921. It was introduced relatively early in France and Nordic countries, but acceptance was much slower in the US, England and Ireland. Price applied for a licence to use the BCG vaccine on an experimental basis in 1936 and first used it at St Ultan's in 1937.[70]

The work of Price and others at St Ultan's produced impressive results: by the 1940s, St Ultan's had reduced its TB mortality from 77 per cent to 28 per cent.[71] Price was appointed as a consultant physician at Newcastle Sanatorium in Dublin and became deeply involved in public health efforts surrounding TB. In 1942 she initiated an exceptionally well-structured programme of public education aimed at early diagnosis and treatment of TB, but encountered significant difficulties owing to the intervention of Dr Charles McQuaid, Catholic Archbishop of Dublin and Primate of Ireland (1940–72). Price was also a member of the Clean Milk Society, aiming to reduce the spread of TB through consumption of contaminated milk.[72] Price's efforts were a significant factor in shaping subsequent governmental efforts to address the problem of TB in Ireland.

In 1948, Dr Noel Browne, Minister for Health (1948–51), formed a national consultative council on TB with Price as chairperson.[73] A National BCG Committee was established, based at St Ultan's Hospital, and a programme of mass BCG vaccination commenced. Finally, Price convinced her medical colleagues of the merits of vaccination.[74]

Overall, Price is best remembered for her extraordinary dedication to the management and eradication of TB, the greatest public health and social problem in early twentieth-century Ireland.[75] During her lifetime, Price developed a strong international reputation as an expert in TB[76] although, following her death, her unique contribution to social medicine in Ireland was largely and tragically forgotten.[77]

From an academic perspective, Price wrote extensively on the subject of TB in journals including the *British Medical Journal*, *Irish Journal of Medical Science* and *Journal of the Irish Free State Medical Union*. In 1942, she published a textbook titled *Tuberculosis in Childhood*, which included a chapter on tuberculous orthopaedic lesions by Henry F. MacAuley.[78] A second edition was published in 1948[79] and positively reviewed in the *Journal of the American Medical Association* in October 1949.[80]

In February 1954, just a year prior to her death, Price published a detailed 'analysis of BCG vaccinations' in the *Irish Journal of Medical Science*, presenting data on 140,697 BCG vaccinations 'performed during a period of four years, July 1949 to July 1953, throughout the Republic of Ireland by the vaccinating teams of the National BCG Committee, St Ultan's Hospital, Dublin'.[81] The data showed 'steady improvement' in vaccination outcomes, which was, 'no doubt, partly attributable to increased all-round efficiency in administration gained by experience'.[82]

Price's work on TB was strongly connected with her work with Lynn at St Ultan's Infant Hospital. The *Irish Times*, in its 'appreciation' of Lynn following her death in September 1955, noted that 'not the least of the achievements of Teach Ultain [St Ultan's] is that it supplied the material, the opportunity and the encouragement for the late Dr Dorothy Price's researches in primary tuberculosis in children. These researches led to the establishment of the BCG unit for inoculation against tuberculosis.'[83]

In 1951, the Executive Committee of the Irish Medical Association nominated Price for the Leon Bernard Foundation prize, awarded by the World Health Organisation for practical achievement in social medicine. The *Irish Times*, in its obituary of Price, described her as 'one of Ireland's most outstanding authorities in the treatment of tuberculosis and a pioneer of BCG vaccination in these islands… Due to Dr Price's foresight and enthusiasm, BCG vaccination was introduced into this country first in 1937'.[84]

Like Price and many other doctors of this era, English, too, was deeply concerned with TB. In 1913, English applied (unsuccessfully) for the post of 'Tuberculosis Officer for Roscommon'.[85] As was the case in many mental hospitals, TB was a key challenge in Ballinasloe throughout English's time there, contributing strongly to morbidity and mortality and necessitating careful planning of new buildings and developments (see Chapter Three).

Like English and Lynn, Price was strongly committed to the Irish nationalist cause and remained an active member of Cumann na mBan throughout her life, despite extensive medical commitments.[86] Like English, Price also opposed the Anglo-Irish Treaty and was a supporter of de Valera.[87] In many of these ways, Price's life and work echo those not only of English and Lynn, but also two other remarkable women doctors of this era, Dr Brigid Lyons Thornton and Dr Eleonora Fleury. Lyons is considered next.

Dr Brigid Lyons Thornton (1898–1987)

Dr Brigid Lyons Thornton was another Irish doctor whose life shared significant similarities with those of English, Lynn and Price. Lyons was born in Northyard, Scramogue, County Roscommon into a staunchly republican family. Her father, Patrick, had fought in the Land War, been arrested and imprisoned.[88] Lyons attended Northyard National School until the age of nine years, when she went to live with her aunt Annie and Annie's husband, Frank McGuinness, in Longford town.

In 1911, Lyons went to boarding school at the Ursuline Convent in Sligo. Lyons enjoyed her schooling in Sligo but also visited Dublin, where she met other relatives who were deeply involved in the nationalist struggle and, especially, Cumann na mBan. In her final year at school in Sligo, Lyons expressed a desire to study medicine and, despite initial surprise, the Ursuline nuns encouraged her warmly.[89] In June 1915, Lyons was successful in her university examination and Irish language interview, and gained a place in University College Galway, commencing in October 1915. During the summer prior to university, Lyons attended Cumann na mBan meetings in Parnell Square in Dublin with her aunt, where she was introduced to many leading members of the organisation, including Lynn.[90]

During her medical studies in Galway, Lyons kept busy with various political and republican activities. She set up a branch of Cumann na mBan and, like English, Lynn and Price, was involved in delivering first-aid lectures, amongst other activities.[91]

On Tuesday of Easter week in 1916, as the Easter Rising was unfolding, Lyons travelled to Dublin where her aunt was involved with Cumann na mBan, supporting the republicans.[92] Lyons, too, joined in the republican effort, starting with making tea and preparing food in the Four Courts, alongside other Cumann na mBan members.[93] Like English and Lynn, Lyons put her medical skills to work too, setting up a first-aid post at a house on Church Street.[94] Lyons also prepared food there, cutting up mutton with a bayonet.[95] Following the republicans' surrender, Lyons was arrested and spent nine days in Kilmainham Gaol.[96]

Following the 1916 Rising, Lyons had to obtain a special permit from British Military authorities to return to Galway, which was under martial law following the Rising in County Galway, led by Mellows. Lyons, now a republican celebrity of sorts, managed to resume her medical studies in Galway. In May 1917, to her great joy, her uncle, Joe McGuinness, was elected as a republican member of parliament.[97] Like English in 1921, McGuinness was in prison at the time of his election in 1917.

Throughout the remainder of her medical studies, Lyons remained highly politically active and deeply connected with republican leaders, especially Michael Collins whom she met at Longford Court in 1918 and who later wrote to her from Sligo prison.[98] There was an interruption to her studies in October 1918, however, when Lyons contracted the Great Flu of 1918–9.[99] Ireland was very badly affected by the global influenza epidemic, which affected some 100 million people worldwide.[100] In Ireland, Lyons was among the 800,000 people infected, of whom 20,000 died.

Lyons, however, recovered and by April 1919 had re-located to Dublin to attend clinical sessions at the Mater Hospital (where English had briefly worked) and completed her medical studies at University College Dublin (the successor to the Catholic University, at which English studied).[101] In parallel with her studies, Lyons remained an active member of Cumann na mBan (University College Dublin branch)[102] and engaged in myriad political activities, including storing republican documents, taking messages for Michael Collins (who trusted her implicitly)[103] and transporting arms for members of the Irish Volunteers in Galway.[104] In April 1921, Lyons played a key role in Collins's unsuccessful attempt to rescue Seán Mac Eoin, a republican soldier and politician, from Mountjoy Prison in Dublin.[105]

Lyons doggedly continued her medical studies. At Mercer's Hospital in Dublin, she encountered and treated casualties from the War of Independence and found, to her surprise, that the hospital's medical and surgical staff had considerable regard for the aspirations of the republicans.[106] On 11 July 1921, a truce in the War of Independence came into effect and on 6 August 1921 Mac Eoin was finally released. Like English, however, Lyons was dismayed at the divisions and bitterness apparent in the subsequent debate over the Anglo-Irish Treaty, which Lyons, unlike English, supported.[107] She was so troubled by the deteriorating political situation that even her success in her final medical examinations in 1922 barely lifted her spirits.[108] In June 1922, as the Civil War developed, Lyons volunteered her services for the pro-Treaty side at the National Army Headquarters in City Hall.[109] During this period Lyons spent time in a first-aid post located on Sackville Street (later O'Connell Street), the same street on which English, on the opposing side, reportedly served with Brugha, at the Hammam Hotel.[110]

Throughout this time, Lyons was also seeking work as a doctor, and, like English, demonstrated an interest in working in asylums. To this end, Lyons applied for a post at Grangegorman Mental Hospital, although another applicant, Dr John Dunne, was successful on that occasion.[111] Dunne went on to a long and distinguished career in Irish psychiatry, eventually becoming RMS of the hospital (1937–65) and president of the Medico-Psychological Association (1955).[112] Following her application to Grangegorman, Collins contacted Lyons asking, in Lyons's words, 'Why didn't you let me know you wanted a job in Grangegorman?'[113] By that point it was too late, however, as Lyons withdrew her application following the death of her uncle.

Lyons met again with Collins not long before his death in 1922 and Collins suggested that she consider working in the Army Medical Services, which were being re-organised by Dr Maurice Hayes.[114] In September 1922 Lyons duly entered the Army Medical Service as a First Lieutenant on a pay of eight shillings a day. As a result, Lyons was the first woman commissioned in the Irish Free State Army.[115]

One of Lyons's tasks during the Civil War was to tend to the medical needs of female political prisoners in Kilmainham Gaol, many of whom were Cumann na mBan members who, unlike Lyons, opposed the Treaty.[116] This was a difficult, complicated assignment for Lyons, tending to prisoners such as Kathleen Clarke, a founder member of Cumann na mBan, and Grace (Gifford) Plunkett, widow of Joseph Plunkett.[117]

In early 1923, Lyons was transferred to work at St Bricin's Military Hospital where her duties included medical administration, for which her previous experience organising elections and engaging in office work had prepared her well.[118] Soon, however, like so many of her countrymen, Lyons contracted TB and was admitted to the Richmond Hospital. In the early 1900s, TB was a major public health problem, accounting for almost 16 per cent of all deaths in Ireland.[119] It was an even bigger problem in mental hospitals, where it accounted for over 25 per cent of deaths.[120] This was similar to the situation in mental hospitals in other countries.[121] English, Lynn, Price and Lyons were all to devote considerable time and effort to combating TB.

During her convalescence, Lyons was summoned to see W.T. Cosgrave, first President of the Executive Council of the Irish Free State (1922–32). Cosgrave offered to lend Lyons £200 from a fund created for individuals who had fallen ill as a result of war activity; the money was to be repaid over time from Lyons's war pension.[122] With this money, Lyons went to Nice in France, a destination suggested as a treatment for TB. There, she met Captain Edward Thornton, an officer in the National Army and fellow-TB patient, with whom she became friendly; he later left the army to train as a barrister and solicitor.

Following further medical advice, Lyons went on to Leysin Fedey in the Swiss Alps, where she was not only treated as a patient but also learned about new treatments for TB from Dr Roulier.[123] Lyons reported positively on her experiences at Leysin Fedey and the next patient sent there was her friend Captain Edward Thornton. Lyons and Thornton would later marry, following their return to Ireland in September 1925.[124] Beforehand, however, Lyons had opportunity to assist medical staff at Leysin Fedey and attend lectures, greatly deepening her knowledge of TB.

Lyons had by now developed a strong interest in public health and in April 1928 began working in the tuberculosis service in Kildare.[125] She was soon moved to Cork and, in September 1929, was appointed permanently to the Dublin Corporation Public Health Service. Like Lynn, Lyons was deeply concerned about children's health, and spent much of her subsequent career as a child welfare paediatrician for Dublin Corporation at the Carnegie Centre in Lord Edward Street.[126]

Throughout her life, Lyons remained engaged in myriad activities in addition to her work for Dublin Corporation. She taught on the Diploma in Public Health course at University College Dublin; was appointed as librarian at the Rotunda Hospital; acted as secretary to the public health section of the Royal Academy of Medicine in Ireland; and became involved with the Medical Benevolent Fund, providing support for doctors and their families in financial difficulties.[127]

Lyons died in 1987 and was buried on Easter Monday, precisely seventy-one years after she had travelled to Dublin to the Four Courts, at the start of the 1916 Easter Rising.

Lyons's life bore many similarities to those of English, Lynn and Price. In the first instance, Lyons was a strongly republican doctor, active in Cumann na mBan and dedicated to the provision of medical support to the republican cause. Like English, Lynn and Price, Lyons's involvement in the republican cause was not, however, limited to medical matters: Lyons transported messages and weapons to republican colleagues, participated in Collins's effort to rescue Mac Eoin from Mountjoy Prison in 1921, and engaged very broadly in many aspects of the republican struggle.

Unlike English and Lynn, Lyons supported the Treaty, and this brought her into conflict with former colleagues from Cumann na mBan. This tension became acutely apparent during the Civil War when Lyons had to tend to female political prisoners in Kilmainham Gaol, many of whom were Cumann na mBan members who, unlike Lyons, opposed the Treaty.[128] Also unlike English and Lynn, Lyons did not enter Dáil Éireann, choosing instead to devote her efforts to work in public health, medicine and paediatrics in the emerging Irish state.[129]

It is interesting that, at one point, Lyons, like English, showed an interest in working in Irish mental hospitals. In the early 1900s, the mental hospitals were vast, complicated institutions urgently in need of medical attention and administrative reform.[130] They also, quite commonly, had strongly republican atmospheres:[131] not only was English practicing both republican politics and medicine at the mental hospital in Ballinasloe, but Grangegorman Mental Hospital, to which Lyons applied, was the workplace of another remarkable figure, Dr Eleonora Fleury, who combined staunch republican activism with highly progressive medical practice. Her extraordinary story is considered next.

Dr Eleonora Fleury (1867–1960)

Eleonora (Norah) Lilian Fleury was born in Manchester in 1867.[132] Her father, Charles Fleury, was a surgeon from a Waterford Anglican family. Fleury studied medicine at the London School of Medicine for Women and the Royal Free

Hospital. Fleury received first-class honours and in 1890 became the first female medical graduate of the Royal University of Ireland.[133] In 1893, Fleury was awarded an MD from the Royal University of Ireland for which she won a gold medal.[134] Fleury went on to work at Homerton (Fever) Hospital in London, the Richmond Asylum in Grangegorman, Dublin (later St Brendan's Hospital) and its sister asylum in Portrane, County Dublin (later St Ita's Hospital).[135]

The Richmond Asylum had been established in 1814 in response to growing evidence of unmet medical and social need amongst the mentally ill.[136] In Dublin, in particular, the patients were often housed in workhouses unsuited to their needs, or wandered the streets in states of destitution. When the Richmond Asylum opened, a Board of Governors was appointed with full powers 'for the regulation, direction and management of themselves and of the said asylum and of all the patients therein and of all and every physician, surgeons, apothecaries, housekeepers, nurse-tenders, and other attendants, officers and servants of what nature and description soever of or belonging to the same'.[137]

From the outset, the Richmond was to employ the 'moral management' paradigm of treatment, emphasising that the doctor should speak rationally with each patient, and the patient should enjoy a healthy diet, exercise frequently and engage in gainful occupation.[138] This relatively enlightened approach persisted for several decades. By 1846, the Richmond had 289 inpatients and the Inspector of Lunatic Asylums in Ireland provided a generally positive assessment:

> It is unnecessary for me to add that the general business [of the asylum] is most satisfactorily performed… The asylum continues to maintain its high character as being one of the best-managed institutions in the country; and also for the great order, regularity, and state of cleanliness in which is it kept.[139]

As the 1800s progressed, however, the Richmond, like the other asylums, expanded at an alarming rate.[140] As a result, official attention shifted from the humane treatment of individual patients to the management of the increasingly complex institutions themselves. By the early 1890s, when Fleury arrived to work there, the Richmond Asylum had almost 1,500 patients resident in accommodation designed for 1,100.[141] In 1893, the 'Inspectors of Lunatics (Ireland)' painted a grim picture:

> During the year no relief has been obtained as regards the overcrowding… It is therefore not to be wondered at that the general health of the institution is far from satisfactory, and that the death-rate, as compared

with other Irish asylums, is high, amounting to 12.5 per cent, the average death rate in similar institutions in this country being 8.3 per cent. Constant outbreaks of zymotic [acute infectious] disease have occurred. Dysentery has for many years past been almost endemic in this institution – seventy-three cases with fourteen deaths occurred last year, and it may be mentioned that in no less than three of these cases secondary abscesses were found in the liver.[142]

It was into this rather bleak environment that Fleury came to work in the 1890s. As was the case with English, Fleury's decision to work in the mental hospitals was an interesting one, and, like English, Fleury was to devote many years of her life to caring for the mentally ill, despite the institutional and therapeutic challenges of the Irish institutions.

Psychiatry had clearly emerged as a profession within medicine as the 1800s had progressed. This process took a significant step forward with the foundation in 1841 of the Association of Medical Officers of Asylums and Hospitals for the Insane, later known as the Medico-Psychological Association (MPA).[143] The purpose of the MPA was to facilitate communication between doctors working in asylums and thus improve patient care. Since its foundation, however, the MPA had admitted only men as members until, in 1893, Fleury's name was put forward for membership. The dramatic proposal to admit a woman was made by Dr Conolly Norman, forward-looking RMS of the Richmond.[144]

Conolly Norman was a popular member of the MPA and would later edit its journal and serve as president.[145] When nominating Fleury, Conolly Norman noted that the female graduates he had met 'were decidedly superior to the average of male graduates'.[146] Predictably, the nomination caused considerable controversy. The president of the MPA, Dr Lindsay of Derby County Asylum, was, however, strongly in favour:

> I cannot see how in common fairness or on what valid ground legally qualified women can be excluded from membership if they wish to join the Association on the same terms and subject to the same rules as men, and do not expect any exceptions to be made in their favour.[147]

In 1894, the rules of the MPA were duly altered at the general meeting and the amendment to admit women passed by twenty-three votes to seven.[148] Fleury thus became the first woman member in 1894 and her paper on 'Agitated Melancholia in Women' was read at the meeting of the MPA's Irish Division in 1895. The precedent set by Fleury was an important one: by 1900, fourteen women had been or were members of the MPA, although it did not have its first female president, Dr A.H.A. Boyle, until 1939.

In the year following her election to the MPA, the *British Medical Journal* announced that Fleury had just been appointed assistant medical officer at the Richmond:

> The Governors of the Richmond Lunatic Asylum, Dublin, have appointed Miss Eleonora L Fleury to be Assistant Medical Officer on the female side of the house. Miss Fleury obtained highest honours with the first Exhibition at the MB Examination, Royal University, Ireland, 1890, and the Gold Medal with the degree of MD in 1892.[149]

Fleury's work involved not only treating patients but also teaching nurses and attendants studying for the newly-established certificate of proficiency in mental nursing.[150] Interestingly, the *Medical Directory* for 1905 records both Fleury and English at the Richmond in that year, with English there as a clinical assistant, shortly after graduating.[151]

Following the death of Conolly Norman in 1908, Fleury was made medical officer in charge of the female house at the Richmond.[152] In 1912, however, when there was a vacancy for a new head of the Richmond's sister asylum in Portrane, Fleury was passed over, as the committee felt it inadvisable to place a woman in such a position. Fleury later became deputy medical superintendent in Portrane.[153]

Like English, Lynn, Price and Lyons, Fleury's medical concerns extended to population health and wellbeing, and, like Lynn, Fleury was especially concerned about the spread of venereal disease in the early 1900s.[154] Fleury was also deeply involved in the nationalist movement, often using the Richmond and Portrane asylums to conceal and assist wounded Republican fugitives. In a Witness Statement supplied to the Bureau of Military History, Eilis, Bean Uí Chonaill of Clontarf (a member of the Cumann na mBan Executive) recounted the 'removal' of several injured Irish Volunteers to safe houses during the War of Independence, including the injured 'Mr Peter Hunt of Sligo' who 'was one of the most "hunted" men of the time'. Eilis, Bean Uí Chonaill reported that 'a cab brought the patient from a house in Prussia Street to the house of Dr Fleury in the Richmond Asylum',[155] and, thus to safety and medical care.

Mrs Mary Flannery Woods of Rathfarnham, another member of Cumann na mBan, confirms Fleury's role:

> Dr Fleury of Portrane Asylum was wonderful. She took a lot of men from me who were suffering from various ailments. She took James Brogan

when he was suffering from bronchitis and again when he was burnt on the railway. Tormey was also burnt on this occasion and was treated by Dr Fleury. How she cared for them these men told me afterwards. She would first look after her mental patients, then the men I had committed to her care and last she would take her own breakfast. She spent her money on cigarettes and comforts for our men… When Free State troops would swoop on the 'Home' the men 'on the run' used go about the grounds and were mistaken, as intended, of course, for mental patients. Mr Cosgrave's Government found out this and took measures to put an end to it – so I was informed but not by Dr Fleury.[156]

More generally, Woods commented that 'the doctors of Dublin were wonderful. I may have forgotten Dr Lynn and others whose names I cannot remember at the moment. Yes, another – Dr Stopford Price.'[157]

As was the case with English, Fleury's activism landed her in trouble with the authorities. On 10 April 1923, Fleury was arrested for treating wounded Republicans at the asylum in Portrane.[158] While in Kilmainham Gaol, Fleury's medical skills proved invaluable, as medical specialists were denied entry to the gaol, despite demonstrated need.[159] Fleury was also interned at the North Dublin Union building which had been requisitioned by the British Military in 1918 as a barracks and transferred to the Irish Free State Army in 1922.[160] In the North Dublin Union internment camp, Fleury joined a group of militant female prisoners who, in May 1923, formed a Prisoners' Council, with Una Gordon as chairperson. Fleury took responsibility (from the prisoners' perspective) for the hospital ward, although there already was an official prison medical officer, Dr Laverty.

Fleury's medical skills were in high demand among the internees. Albinia Lucy Brodrick, for example, was arrested on 1 May 1923 in Kerry, having acquired a gunshot wound to her leg while tending to wounded Republicans in Listowel.[161] On arrival in the North Dublin Union, Brodrick promptly went on hunger strike and refused medical care from Dr Laverty, but permitted Fleury to tend to her, as a fellow-internee.

The prisoners at the North Dublin Union were extremely vocal and active, protesting strongly against their conditions. Some escaped over the walls into the neighbouring Broadstone railway station. In May 1923, a second Prisoners' Council was elected, with Fleury staying on as medical officer with responsibility for the hospital ward.[162] By this time, the hospital ward had accommodation for twenty patients, who presented a broad range of medical problems, including epilepsy, scarlet fever, scabies and lice.[163] Hygiene was a constant problem and Fleury worked with the prison medical officer to maintain hygiene among the internees.

In June 1923, however, the governor of the internment camp refused to sanction the carrying of coal to the hospital ward and Fleury withdrew her services in protest.[164] Some of the prisoners went on hunger strike. Early the following month, on 7 July 1923, Fleury was released and promptly denounced conditions in the North Dublin Union in a strongly-worded article in *Irish Nation (Éire)*, a Republican paper. Fleury wrote that the internment camp was filthy, 'scabies and lice were a problem' and 'illnesses like scarlet fever, chickenpox and smallpox were a cause for concern'.[165] Fleury's article resulted in a formal inspection of the North Dublin Union, which strongly supported Fleury's concerns.

Following her long, distinguished medical career, Fleury lived, for most of her retirement, at 239 Upper Rathmines Road in Dublin. Like Lynn, she remained physically active all her life. Fleury died in 1960 and is buried in Mount Jerome Cemetery in Harold's Cross.

Overall, Fleury and English had much in common: both were early female medical graduates who devoted their careers to the mentally ill, both worked at the Richmond Asylum in Dublin, both were nationalist activists, and both were incarcerated at various points; neither married. Fleury made a particular contribution to the advancement of women in psychiatry by becoming the first female member of the MPA in 1894 and, thus, the first female psychiatrist in Ireland or Great Britain. In doing so, Fleury paved the way for future female psychiatrists, such as English, who was also active in the MPA.[166]

Unlike English, Fleury was not elected to Dáil Éireann, but, like English, she readily recognised the usefulness of the large asylum setting to further her political aims. To this extent at least, for both Fleury and English, the fight for Irish freedom was inseparable from their working and personal lives.

Like Lynn, Price and Lyons, Fleury and English both combined progressive medical practice with acute social conscience, political awareness and republican activism. These women made these remarkable contributions at a time when Ireland was undergoing a period of exceptionally rapid political change and there appeared to be genuine opportunities to effect political, social and (possibly) medical reform, for the betterment of all.

Conclusion

English, Lynn, Price, Lyons and Fleury all made significant contributions to Irish medicine and politics in various ways. From a scientific and medical perspective, their names belong with those of a number of other Irish women who made substantial contributions to science and medicine during this period.[167] These include, amongst others, the 'fabulous Boole sisters', daughters of George Boole, mathematician and logician, and Mary Everest, educational psychologist. This remarkable family included Alicia Boole Stott, a distinguished mathematician, Lucy Boole, the first woman professor of chemistry in Britain, and Ethel Lilian Voynich, a best-selling novelist and revolutionary.[168]

Other Irish women pioneers of this era included Alice Everett, a physicist, and Annie Dill Russell, a renowned observer of solar eclipses.[169] Aleen Cust, born in Tipperary, was the first women veterinarian in Ireland and Britain, and Alice Perry, born in Galway, was the first woman engineering graduate in Ireland and Britain.[170] Irish geology also benefitted from the contributions of female pioneers such as Sydney Mary Thompson, Mary K. Andrews, Doris Livesley Reynolds and Veronica Conroy Burns.[171]

English was one of very few progressive woman doctors working within the asylum system over this period; others included Fleury, who also shared English's dedication to advancing Ireland's nationalist cause. Emily Winifred Dickson was another comparable figure who worked in asylums and shared English's concern with public health, although Dickson worked in the English asylum system and for shorter periods than English. Dickson had graduated with first-class honours from the Royal College of Surgeons in Ireland in 1893 and later worked at Rainhill Mental Hospital in northern England.[172] Like English, Dickson lectured extensively, was involved in the Irish Women's National Health Association[173] and was deeply concerned with public health, especially among the socially excluded.[174]

Although Dickson married in 1899, her views on women doctors getting married may well have been shared by English, who did not. Kelly notes that in 1899 Dickson delivered a paper at a meeting of the Alexandra College Guild titled 'Medicine as a Profession for Women' and was asked about marriage:[175]

> Dr Dickson, in the course of her reply, said it was impossible to make any general rules to marriage. That was a question that every person had to settle for herself. *(Laughter.)* If a woman who had spent the best years of her life in preparing for a medical degree was bound on entering the married state to give up the medical profession it would tend to lower the status of the married state. For her part she thought a woman should not give up the medical profession for the profession of marriage unless she liked the latter profession better. *(Laughter).*[176]

English clearly chose to devote her life to her political activities and the medical profession, rather than 'the profession of marriage'. The reforms that English subsequently championed at Ballinasloe were important ones, and her tireless campaigning for legal reform at national level was also recognised in the year following her death, in the Mental Treatment Act 1945 (see Chapter Five).

What is truly remarkable about English, Lynn, Price, Lyons and Fleury, however, is the fact that all five of these doctors combined sustained political activism with progressive medical practice, and many of their contributions remained relevant to Irish public health even several decades after their deaths. More than half a century after the death of Lynn, for example, her approach to child healthcare was readily evoked in discussions regarding the development of a new national children's hospital in Dublin.[177] In 2011, Dr Mary Henry, a former independent member of Seanad Éireann, wrote that it was 'a wonderful idea to name the new children's hospital after Dr Kathleen Lynn' who had great 'plans in the 1930s for a large children's hospital':

> Her plans did not find favour with Archbishop John Charles McQuaid. He was very important in scuppering this initiative – non-Catholic and Catholic children were to be cared for together and of this he did not approve. Since the new hospital will care for and cherish all the children of the nation equally and together, it would be fitting to see her initiative of over seventy years ago remembered.[178]

Lynn's pragmatic, progressive and enduring approach to health care was also echoed in various ways in the work of English, Price, Lyons and Fleury. While English and Fleury focused their medical work on the mentally ill, they were also, like Lynn, Price and Lyons, deeply concerned about the medical and social wellbeing of the disadvantaged, and consistently associated this concern with the need for political and social change. The decision of these women to enter medicine in the first instance was likely linked, at least in part, to their personal awareness of health and social problems during their childhoods. Their continued awareness of the social context of medicine was likely deepened by their medical training, growing political awareness, experiences in the practice of their profession, and contacts with other woman practitioners.

Price, for example, was deeply influenced by Dr Ella Webb, another early medical graduate (1904) and political activist in Dublin.[179] Webb let Price 'go down and help her in her slum dispensary on Tuesday evenings and shows what simply wonderful things a person can do besides doctoring'.[180] More broadly, Price's work on TB drew attention to concerns about the links between TB, malnutrition and social conditions, both in the general population and, especially, among children.[181]

Similar themes are apparent in the work of Lyons and English, as exemplified by English's contribution to the Irish Catholic Truth Society Conference at the

Mansion House in Dublin in 1921. The Catholic Truth Society was founded in 1868 by Cardinal Herbert Vaughan, an English prelate of the Roman Catholic Church. The Society's primary role was to publish Catholic literature such as prayer-books, spiritual reading and apologetics. The Catholic Truth Society of Ireland was founded in 1899 and their 1921 conference, at which English spoke, heard discussions on a range of topics including 'home-life, intellectualism and mixed marriages' (i.e. marriages of Catholics with Protestants).[182]

There was particular opposition to mixed marriages. 'Miss E.M. O'Neill, BA, of Derry', for example, 'read a paper on "Catholic Home Life"', arguing that 'the spirit of every Irish Catholic household was fundamentally religious':

> Never did the Irish people need those holy influences more than at present. The intellectualism of the present day was very much of a 'devil's advocate'. It had the subtlety of satanic cunning and the specious arguments of the Father of Lies… The absolute essential to a Catholic home was a thoroughly Catholic atmosphere, and that presupposed Catholic parentage. The beautiful bond of family affection was, she said, perfect only when all the members of the family lived and loved in the common practice of the true faith.[183]

Not everyone, however, agreed with the supreme importance that O'Neill attached to Catholic home-life. English spoke out:

> Dr Ada English, MP, held the view that there could be a too intensive cultivation of home life to the exclusion of other matters. There were social and national movements which necessarily drew people from the home life, and they should be prepared to take their share in these movements, and ready to encounter and counter opposition by the practical application of the teachings of their faith in matters of everyday life. She advocated decent housing for the working classes for it was impossible that people who were condemned to dwell in wretched, crowded insanitary houses could cherish or practice any high ideals either of religion or nationality.[184]

Lynn held similar views, strongly linking health with social conditions and the need for political change. In 1919, for example, Pádraig Pearse's play 'The Singer' was staged at the Abbey Theatre in support of St Ultan's Hospital and Lynn gave a speech clearly linking infant health with social conditions.[185] She stated that 'infant mortality was in direct proportion to the amount of money that the parents had, and it was the duty of every man and woman who had money enough for simple necessities of life and something over to give that surplus to assist children who, without their aid, must inevitably perish'.[186]

Lynn's concerns extended from infant's health to venereal disease, from the influenza pandemic to the provision of public lavatories for women in Dublin's city centre.[187] In short, Lynn was concerned with both the health of the individual and the social environment in which that health was to be achieved and enjoyed. Similar concerns informed the work and outlooks of Price, Lyons and English.

Both Lynn and English saw the achievement of an Ireland that was free, prosperous and at peace as critical for attaining their desired health and social goals. In 1922, during the Dáil debate on the Anglo-Irish Treaty, English spoke of the need for a balance between the political agitation for Irish freedom and the desire for 'quietness and peace':

> The country is not for this Treaty, the country is out for peace. The country wants peace and desires peace. So do we. We all want peace, but we want a peace which will be a real peace and a lasting peace and a peace based on honour and on friendship and a peace which we can keep, a peace that we can put our names to and stand by. That is the sort of peace the country wants, and it is only because the country is misled into believing that this Treaty gives such a peace that the country wants it. The country wants no peace which gives away the independence of Ireland and destroys the Republic which has been established by the will of the Irish people *(hear, hear)*. We have had painted for us in various lurid colours the terrors of war and the desire of the people for quietness and peace. Well, peace is a good thing, but in the days of the famine the people were also told that they should be peaceful and submissive and quiet, and accept what the English chose to give them – the rotten potatoes – and let the corn and food be exported out of the country. There were people then, Republicans and Revolutionists, who encouraged the people to fight for the country in spite of the men with the streak, and free themselves and keep the food in the country. But some of the influences that are working against the country to-day were working against it then and advised peace. They got peace – and death and famine. You can lose more men – their bodies as well as their souls – by an ignoble peace than by fighting for just rights *(cheers)*.[188]

'Fighting for just rights' was a key concern for English in her medical career too, not least because she was working in asylums and mental hospitals at a time when reform was urgently needed. Most worryingly, the over-crowding, which had commenced in the early 1800s, seemed to be continuing inexorably,[189] despite careful consideration of the matter by the Conference of the Irish

Asylums Committee in 1903[190] and the establishment of no fewer than three official commissions of inquiry between 1906 and 1910.[191] Despite this level of professional and governmental concern, conditions remained extremely difficult throughout the 1920s. In 1924, Edward Boyd Barrett SJ wrote an outspoken article in *Studies*, an 'Irish quarterly review', pointing out that 'our asylums are in a bad way'[192] and recommending that:

> There should be a strong public demand for immediate reform of the asylum system, and the complete segregation and scientific treatment of curable cases should be insisted upon. Suitable asylums should be built – healthy, bright, beautiful homes, where patients would be enticed by every art to renew their interests in things. Nerve clinics should be opened in every populous district, where advice and treatment should be available for ordinary cases of nerve trouble and incipient insanity.[193]

There was widespread acknowledgement of the need for these kinds of reforms and in 1927 this was further underlined by the *Commission on the Relief of the Sick and Destitute Poor, including Insane Poor,* which recommended the establishment of outpatient clinics and auxiliary psychiatric hospitals in order to reduce pressure on existing mental hospitals.[194] Reform of mental health system was, however, to take much longer, and, despite English's urgings, revised mental health legislation was not introduced until 1945, a year after her death.[195]

By the time of her death, however, it was already apparent that English had made significant contributions to Irish medicine (especially mental health services) in addition to her participation in the republican cause. In these ways, English's life and career ultimately demonstrated their most important overlap with those of Lynn, Price, Lyons and Fleury: all contributed significantly to *both* medicine and the republican struggle in the emerging Irish state.

Perhaps the greatest single overlap between the lives and careers of these five remarkable women lay in the vision that they shared of a health service that would recognise the social landscape in which ill-health develops and is treated, and the connection they saw between building an effective health system and building a country that was equitable, just and free.

To this extent, these women were living embodiments of the views of Rudolf Virchow, the German pathologist and politician, who declared that 'medicine is a social science, and politics nothing but medicine on a large scale'.[196] The lives and contributions of English, Lynn, Price, Lyons and Fleury certainly supported the truth of Virchow's statement, and their pioneering work demonstrated the power of combining medicine with revolutionary politics at a time of exceptional challenge and opportunity in Irish history.

Notes

1. Ferriter, *The Transformation of Ireland 1900–2000*, pp.185, 399–404, 422; R. Barrington, *Health, Medicine and Politics in Ireland, 1900–1970* (Dublin: Institute of Public Administration, 1987), pp.24–136.
2. Ó hÓgartaigh, *Kathleen Lynn: Irishwoman, Patriot, Doctor* (Dublin: Irish Academic Press, 2006), p.6.
3. McNamara and Mooney, *Women in Parliament: 1918–2000* (Dublin: Wolfhound Press, 2000), p.87.
4. M. Ó hÓgartaigh, '"Is there any need of you?" Women in medicine in Ireland and Australia', *Australian Journal of Irish Studies*, 4 (2004), pp.162–71.
5. Ó hÓgartaigh, *Kathleen Lynn: Irishwoman, Patriot, Doctor*, pp.11–12.
6. D. Kelly *Between the Lines of History* (Ballinasloe: Declan Kelly, 2000), p.25.
7. Ó hÓgartaigh, *Kathleen Lynn: Irishwoman, Patriot, Doctor*, p.13.
8. Ibid., p.19.
9. Mac Curtain, *Ariadne's Thread: Writing Women into Irish History* (Galway: Arlen House, 2008), p.89.
10. J. Cowell, *A Noontide Blazing: Brigid Lyons Thornton – Rebel, Soldier, Doctor* (Dublin: Currach Press, 2005), p.39.
11. *Irish Times*, 15 September 1955.
12. R.M. Fox, 'The Irish Citizen Army', in B. Ó Conchubhair (ed.), *Dublin's Fighting Story 1916–1921, Told By The Men Who Made It* (Dublin: Mercier Press, 2009), pp.52–9; Ó hÓgartaigh, *Quiet Revolutionaries: Irish Women in Education, Medicine and Sport, 1861–1964*, p.94; Ó hÓgartaigh, *Kathleen Lynn: Irishwoman, Patriot, Doctor*, p.21; Eichacker, *Irish Republican Women in America: Lecture Tours, 1916–1925*, p.9.
13. Kelly, *Between the Lines of History*, p.25; McNamara and Mooney, *Women in Parliament: 1918–2000*, p.79.
14. McNamara and Mooney, *Women in Parliament: 1918–2000*, p.87; Matthews, *Renegades: Irish Republican Women, 1900–1922* (Cork: Mercier Press, 2010), p.82.
15. Ó hÓgartaigh, *Kathleen Lynn: Irishwoman, Patriot, Doctor*, pp.23–6.
16. Matthews, *Renegades*, p.121.
17. Ibid., p.127.
18. Matthews, *Renegades*, p.339.
19. McCoole, *No Ordinary Women: Irish Female Activists in the Revolutionary Years, 1900–1923*, p.36; Meenan, *Cecilia Street: The Catholic University School of Medicine, 1855–1931* (Dublin: Gill and Macmillan, 1987), p.95.
20. R.M. Fox, 'Citizen Army posts', in B. Ó Conchubhair (ed.), *Dublin's Fighting Story 1916–1921, Told By The Men Who Made It* (Dublin: Mercier Press, 2009), pp.107–17; Mac Curtain, *Ariadne's Thread*, p.216; A. Mac Lellan. 'Revolutionary doctors', in M. Mulvihill (ed.), *Lab Coats and Lace: The Lives and Legacies of Inspiring Irish Women Scientists and Pioneers* (Dublin: Women in Technology and Science, 2009), pp.86–101.
21. McCoole, *No Ordinary Women: Irish Female Activists in the Revolutionary Years, 1900–1923*, p.45.
22. McNamara and Mooney, *Women in Parliament: 1918–2000*, p.79; *Irish Press*, 28 January 1944; *East Galway Democrat*, 29 January 1944.

23. Matthews, *Renegades*, p.155; McNamara and Mooney, *Women in Parliament: 1918–2000*, p.88. See also: McCarthy, *Cumann na mBan and the Irish Revolution*, p.72; Eichacker, *Irish Republican Women in America: Lecture Tours, 1916–1925*, pp.13–14, 211.

24. R.M. Fox, 'How the women helped', in B. Ó Conchubhair (ed.), *Dublin's Fighting Story 1916–1921, Told By The Men Who Made It* (Dublin: Mercier Press, 2009), pp.395–405; A. Clare, *Unlikely Rebels: The Gifford Girls and the Fight for Irish Freedom* (Dublin: Mercier Press, 2011), p.190.

25. Ó hÓgartaigh, *Kathleen Lynn: Irishwoman, Patriot, Doctor*, p.32. See also: McCoole, *No Ordinary Women: Irish Female Activists in the Revolutionary Years, 1900–1923*, pp.56–7.

26. Matthews, *Renegades*, p.157.

27. Clare, *Unlikely Rebels: The Gifford Girls and the Fight for Irish Freedom*, p.199; McCoole, *No Ordinary Women: Irish Female Activists in the Revolutionary Years, 1900–1923*, p.65; Ó hÓgartaigh, *Kathleen Lynn: Irishwoman, Patriot, Doctor*, p.34.

28. Ó hÓgartaigh, *Kathleen Lynn: Irishwoman, Patriot, Doctor*, p.42.

29. Matthews, *Renegades*, p.205.

30. J. Knirk, *Women of the Dáil: Gender, Republicanism and the Anglo-Irish Treaty* (Dublin: Irish Academic Press, 2006), pp.16–17; M. Ward, 'Times of transition: Republican women, feminism and political representation', in L. Ryan and M. Ward (eds), *Irish Women and Nationalism: Soldiers, New Women and Wicked Hags* (Dublin: Irish Academic Press, 2004), pp.184–201.

31. Ó hÓgartaigh, *Kathleen Lynn: Irishwoman, Patriot, Doctor*, p.47.

32. Matthews, *Renegades*, p.292. See also: Matthews, *Dissidents: Irish Republican Women, 1923–1941*, p.31.

33. Clancy, *Contesting Politics: Women in Ireland, North and South*, p.206.

34. Quoted in: Ó hÓgartaigh, *Kathleen Lynn: Irishwoman, Patriot, Doctor*, p.52.

35. Matthews, *Renegades*, p.253.

36. Ó hÓgartaigh, *Kathleen Lynn: Irishwoman, Patriot, Doctor*, p.52.

37. Matthews, *Dissidents*, pp.188–9.

38. *Irish Times*, 22 January 1929.

39. Ibid.

40. Matthews, *Renegades*, p.221. See also: McNamara and Mooney, *Women in Parliament: 1918–2000*, p.88.

41. McNamara and Mooney, *Women in Parliament: 1918–2000*, p.88.

42. Mac Lellan, *Lab Coats and Lace: The Lives and Legacies of Inspiring Irish Women Scientists and Pioneers*, p.95.

43. Ó hÓgartaigh, *Kathleen Lynn: Irishwoman, Patriot, Doctor*, pp.75–7.

44. McNamara and Mooney, *Women in Parliament: 1918–2000*, p.89.

45. Ó hÓgartaigh, *Kathleen Lynn: Irishwoman, Patriot, Doctor*, p.93.

46. *Irish Times*, 31 May 1913.

47. Ó hÓgartaigh, *Kathleen Lynn: Irishwoman, Patriot, Doctor*, p.139.

48. *Irish Times*, 16 September 1955.

49. Ibid.

50. Kelly, *Between the Lines of History*, p.25.

51. Ó hÓgartaigh, *Kathleen Lynn: Irishwoman, Patriot, Doctor*, p.19.

52. Matthews, *Renegades*, pp.11, 201–2.

53. Ibid., pp.188–9.

54. M. Mulholland, *The Politics and Relationships of Kathleen Lynn* (Dublin: The Woodfield Press, 2002), pp.16–18.

55. A. Mac Lellan, 'Dr Dorothy Price and the eradication of TB in Ireland', *Irish Medical News*, 19 May 2008. Mac Lellan, A., *Dorothy Stopford Price: Rebel Doctor* (Sallins, Co. Kildare: Irish Academic Press, 2014).

56. M. Ó hÓgartaigh. 'Dorothy Stopford Price and the elimination of childhood tuberculosis' in J. Augusteijn (ed.), *Ireland in the 1930s: New Perspectives* (Dublin: Four Courts Press, 1999), pp.67–82. See also: Ó hÓgartaigh, *Kathleen Lynn: Irishwoman, Patriot, Doctor*, p.74.

57. Matthews, *Renegades*, pp.22–3.

58. Ibid., pp.99, 104, 107 and 218.

59. Ó hÓgartaigh, *Ireland in the 1930s: New Perspectives*, p.107.

60. A. Mac Lellan, 'Dr Dorothy Price and the eradication of TB in Ireland', *Irish Medical News*, 19 May 2008.

61. Ó hÓgartaigh, *Ireland in the 1930s: New Perspectives*, p.107.

62. L. Ó Broin, *Protestant Nationalists in Revolutionary Ireland: The Stopford Connection* (Dublin: Goldenbridge, 1985), p.173.

63. Ó hÓgartaigh, *Quiet Revolutionaries: Irish Women in Education, Medicine and Sport, 1861–1964*, pp.100–1.

64. M. Ó hÓgartaigh. 'Dorothy Stopford Price and the elimination of childhood tuberculosis' in J. Augusteijn (ed.), *Ireland in the 1930s*, pp.67–82.

65. Mac Lellan, *Lab Coats and Lace: The Lives and Legacies of Inspiring Irish Women Scientists and Pioneers*, p.91.

66. Ó hÓgartaigh, *Ireland in the 1930s: New Perspectives*, p.109. See also: B. Kelly, 'The history of medicine', *Irish Medical News*, 8 August 2010.

67. *Irish Press*, 28 January 1944; *East Galway Democrat*, 29 January 1944; McNamara and Mooney, *Women in Parliament: 1918–2000*, p.79.

68. *Irish Times*, 1 February 1954.

69. A. Mac Lellan, 'Dr Dorothy Price and the eradication of TB in Ireland', *Irish Medical News*, 19 May 2008.

70. Ibid.

71. Ó hÓgartaigh, *Quiet Revolutionaries: Irish Women in Education, Medicine and Sport, 1861–1964*, p. 102.

72. Ibid., p.115.

73. Mac Lellan, *Lab Coats and Lace: The Lives and Legacies of Inspiring Irish Women Scientists and Pioneers*, p.99.

74. Ó hÓgartaigh, *Kathleen Lynn: Irishwoman, Patriot, Doctor*, p.133.

75. B. Kelly, 'Female pioneers', *Irish Medical News*, 27 April 2009.

76. Ó hÓgartaigh, *Kathleen Lynn: Irishwoman, Patriot, Doctor*, p.122.

77. Mac Lellan, *Lab Coats and Lace: The Lives and Legacies of Inspiring Irish Women Scientists and Pioneers*, p.99.

78. D. Stopford Price and H.F. MacAuley, *Tuberculosis in Childhood* (Bristol: John Wright, 1942).

79. D. Stopford Price and H.F. MacAuley, *Tuberculosis in Childhood (Second Edition)*

(Bristol: John Wright, 1948).

80. Anonymous, 'Book Notice: Tuberculosis in Children by Dorothy Stopford Price, MD', *Journal of the American Medical Association*, 140, 16 (1949), p.1308.
81. D.S. Price, 'Analysis of BCG vaccinations', *Irish Journal of Medical Science*, 29, 2 (February 1954), pp.56–64.
82. Dorothy S. Price, 'Analysis of BCG vaccinations', *Irish Journal of Medical Science*, 29, 2 (February 1954), pp.56–64.
83. *Irish Times*, 16 September 1955.
84. *Irish Times*, 1 February 1954.
85. *Irish Times*, 31 May 1913.
86. Witness Statement (Number 1,752) of Mrs McCarvill (Eileen McGrane) (Dublin: Bureau of Military History, 1913-21, File Number S.1434), p.12.
87. Ó hÓgartaigh, *Quiet Revolutionaries: Irish Women in Education, Medicine and Sport, 1861–1964*, p.101.
88. Cowell, *A Noontide Blazing: Brigid Lyons Thornton – Rebel, Soldier, Doctor*, p.17.
89. Ibid., p.36.
90. Ibid., p.39.
91. Ibid., p.47.
92. Mac Lellan, *Lab Coats and Lace: The Lives and Legacies of Inspiring Irish Women Scientists and Pioneers*, p.89.
93. Cowell, *A Noontide Blazing: Brigid Lyons Thornton – Rebel, Soldier, Doctor*, p.62.
94. McCoole, *No Ordinary Women: Irish Female Activists in the Revolutionary Years, 1900–1923*, p.40.
95. Mac Lellan, *Lab Coats and Lace: The Lives and Legacies of Inspiring Irish Women Scientists and Pioneers*, p.90.
96. McCoole, *No Ordinary Women: Irish Female Activists in the Revolutionary Years, 1900–1923*, p.49; Cowell, *A Noontide Blazing: Brigid Lyons Thornton – Rebel, Soldier, Doctor*, pp.91–95; Clare, *Unlikely Rebels: The Gifford Girls and the Fight for Irish Freedom*, p.170; Mac Lellan, *Lab Coats and Lace: The Lives and Legacies of Inspiring Irish Women Scientists and Pioneers*, p.90.
97. Cowell, *A Noontide Blazing: Brigid Lyons Thornton – Rebel, Soldier, Doctor*, pp.119–120.
98. Ibid., pp.136–138.
99. Ibid., pp.144–146.
100. C. Foley, *The Last Irish Plague: The Great Flu Epidemic in Ireland, 1918–19* (Dublin: Irish Academic Press, 2011).
101. Cowell, *A Noontide Blazing: Brigid Lyons Thornton – Rebel, Soldier, Doctor*, p.162.
102. Witness Statement (Number 1,752) of Mrs McCarvill (Eileen McGrane) (Dublin: Bureau of Military History, 1913-21, File Number S.1434), p.12.
103. Mac Lellan, *Lab Coats and Lace: The Lives and Legacies of Inspiring Irish Women Scientists and Pioneers*, p.91.
104. McCoole, *No Ordinary Women: Irish Female Activists in the Revolutionary Years, 1900–1923*, p.78; Cowell, *A Noontide Blazing: Brigid Lyons Thornton – Rebel, Soldier, Doctor*, pp.163–4.
105. Cowell, *A Noontide Blazing: Brigid Lyons Thornton – Rebel, Soldier, Doctor*, pp.187–98.
106. Ibid., p.169.

107. McCoole, *No Ordinary Women: Irish Female Activists in the Revolutionary Years, 1900–1923*, p.93.
108. Mac Lellan, *Lab Coats and Lace: The Lives and Legacies of Inspiring Irish Women Scientists and Pioneers*, p.90; Cowell, *A Noontide Blazing: Brigid Lyons Thornton – Rebel, Soldier, Doctor*, pp.221–2.
109. Cowell, *A Noontide Blazing: Brigid Lyons Thornton – Rebel, Soldier, Doctor*, p.225.
110. *Irish Press*, 28 January 1944; McNamara and Mooney, *Women in Parliament: 1918–2000*, p.79; Clarke, 'English, Adeline ('Ada')', in J. McGuire and J. Quinn (eds), *Dictionary of Irish Biography: From the Earliest Times to the Year 2002 (Volume 3, D-F)* (Cambridge: Royal Irish Academy and Cambridge University Press, 2009), pp.626–7.
111. Cowell, *A Noontide Blazing: Brigid Lyons Thornton – Rebel, Soldier, Doctor*, p.227.
112. J. Dunne, 'Survey of modern physical methods of treatment for mental illness carried out in Grangegorman Mental Hospital', *Journal of the Medical Association of Eire*, 27, 157 (1950), pp. 4–9; J. Dunne, 'The contribution of the physical sciences to psychological medicine', *Journal of Mental Science*, 102, 427 (1956), pp.209–20; B.D. Kelly, 'Physical sciences and psychological medicine: the legacy of Prof John Dunne', *Irish Journal of Psychological Medicine*, 22, 2 (2005), pp.67–72. See also: Reynolds, *Grangegorman: Psychiatric Care in Dublin since 1815*.
113. Cowell, *A Noontide Blazing: Brigid Lyons Thornton – Rebel, Soldier, Doctor*, p.227.
114. Ibid., pp.228–230.
115. McCarthy, *Cumann na mBan and the Irish Revolution*, p.220.
116. McCoole, *No Ordinary Women: Irish Female Activists in the Revolutionary Years, 1900–1923*, p.107–108.
117. Cowell, *A Noontide Blazing: Brigid Lyons Thornton – Rebel, Soldier, Doctor*, pp.231–232.
118. Ibid., pp.235–6.
119. G. Jones, 'The Campaign Against Tuberculosis in Ireland, 1899–1914', in E. Malcolm and G. Jones (eds), *Medicine, Disease and the State in Ireland, 1650–1940* (Cork: Cork University Press, 1999), pp.158–76.
120. Finnane, *Insanity and the Insane in Post-Famine Ireland*, p.137.
121. P. McCandless, 'Curative asylum, custodial hospital: the South Carolina Lunatic Asylum and State Hospital, 1828–1920', in R. Porter and D. Wright (eds), *The Confinement of the Insane: International Perspectives, 1800–1965* (Cambridge: Cambridge University Press, 2003), pp.173–92.
122. Mac Lellan, *Lab Coats and Lace: The Lives and Legacies of Inspiring Irish Women Scientists and Pioneers*, p.100; Cowell, *A Noontide Blazing: Brigid Lyons Thornton – Rebel, Soldier, Doctor*, p.238.
123. Cowell, *A Noontide Blazing: Brigid Lyons Thornton – Rebel, Soldier, Doctor*, pp.242–4.
124. Mac Lellan, *Lab Coats and Lace: The Lives and Legacies of Inspiring Irish Women Scientists and Pioneers*, p.100.
125. Cowell, *A Noontide Blazing: Brigid Lyons Thornton – Rebel, Soldier, Doctor*, pp.246–7.
126. Mac Lellan, *Lab Coats and Lace: The Lives and Legacies of Inspiring Irish Women Scientists and Pioneers*, pp.100–1.
127. Cowell, *A Noontide Blazing: Brigid Lyons Thornton – Rebel, Soldier, Doctor*, pp.253–254.

128. McCoole, *No Ordinary Women: Irish Female Activists in the Revolutionary Years, 1900–1923*, p.107–108.
129. B. Kelly, 'The history of medicine', *Irish Medical News*, 8 August 2010.
130. E. Boyd Barrett, 'Modern psycho-therapy and our asylums', *Studies*, 13, 49 (March 1924), pp.9–43.
131. Cox, *Negotiating Insanity in the Southeast of Ireland, 1820–1900*, p.17.
132. A. Collins, 'Eleonora Fleury captured', *British Journal of Psychiatry*, 203, 1 (2013), p.5.
133. M. Ó hÓgartaigh, '"Is there any need of you?"Women in medicine in Ireland and Australia', *Australian Journal of Irish Studies*, 4 (2004), pp.162–71. See also: Kelly, *Irish Women in Medicine, c.1880s–1920s: Origins, Education and Careers*, p.87.
134. Anonymous. 'Medical news', *British Medical Journal*, 1, 1786 (1895), p.679; Anonymous. 'Erratum', *British Medical Journal*, 1, 1787 (1895), p.738.
135. Ó hÓgartaigh, *Quiet Revolutionaries: Irish Women in Education, Medicine and Sport, 1861–1964*, p.147.
136. Reynolds, *Grangegorman: Psychiatric Care in Dublin since 1815*, pp.20–30.
137. B.D. Kelly, 'One hundred years ago: the Richmond Asylum, Dublin in 1907', *Irish Journal of Psychological Medicine*, 24, 3 (September 2007), pp.108–14.
138. Reynolds, *Grangegorman: Psychiatric Care in Dublin since 1815*, pp.16–19.
139. Inspector of Lunatic Asylums in Ireland. *Report of the District, Local, and Private Lunatic Asylums in Ireland, 1846 (With Appendices)* (Dublin: Alexander Thom for Her Majesty's Stationery Office, 1847), p.19.
140. Robins, *Fools and Mad*, pp.128–42; B.D. Kelly, 'Mental health law in Ireland, 1821 to 1902: building the asylums', *Medico-Legal Journal*, 76, 1 (2008), pp.19–25; B.D. Kelly, 'Mental health law in Ireland, 1821 to 1902: dealing with the "increase of insanity in Ireland"', *Medico-Legal Journal*, 7, 1 (2008), pp.26–33.
141. Inspectors of Lunatics (Ireland), 1893; p.9.
142. Ibid.
143. Bewley, *Madness to Mental Illness: A History of the Royal College of Psychiatrists*, p.10.
144. Reynolds, *Grangegorman: Psychiatric Care in Dublin since 1815*, pp.152–3.
145. Bewley, *Madness to Mental Illness: A History of the Royal College of Psychiatrists*, p.26.
146. S. Floate and Harcourt Williams, M. 'Sketches from the history of psychiatry: "an innovation, a revolution" – the admission of women members to the Medico-Psychological Association', *Psychiatric Bulletin*, 15, 1 (1991), pp.28–30.
147. J.M. Lindsay, 'Presidential address delivered at the Fifty-Second Annual Meeting of the Medico-Psychological Association, held at the Palace Hotel, Buxton, 28 July, 1893', *Journal of Mental Science*, 39, 167 (1893), pp.473–91.
148. Bewley, *Madness to Mental Illness: A History of the Royal College of Psychiatrists*, p.27.
149. Anonymous. 'Medical news', *British Medical Journal*, 1, 1786 (1895), p.679. In fact, Fleury received her MD in 1893 and not 1892, as the *British Medical Journal* admitted the following week. (Anonymous. 'Erratum', *British Medical Journal*, 1, 1787 (1895), p.738).
150. Reynolds, *Grangegorman: Psychiatric Care in Dublin since 1815*, p.189.
151. *Medical Directory for 1905* (London: J. & A. Churchill, 1905), pp.1414, 1417.
152. Reynolds, *Grangegorman: Psychiatric Care in Dublin since 1815*, p.210.
153. Ibid., p.229.

154. Matthews, *Renegade*, pp.208–9.

155. Witness Statement (Number 568) of Eilis, Bean Uí Chonaill (Dublin: Bureau of Military History, 1913–21, File Number S.1846), pp.53–4.

156. Witness Statement (Number 624) of Mrs Mary Flannery Woods (Dublin: Bureau of Military History, 1913–21, File Number S.1901), pp.28–9.

157. Witness Statement (Number 624) of Mrs Mary Flannery Woods (Dublin: Bureau of Military History, 1913–21, File Number S.1901), p.57.

158. Matthews, *Dissidents: Irish Republican Women, 1923–1941*, p.90.

159. McCoole, *No Ordinary Women: Irish Female Activists in the Revolutionary Years, 1900–1923*, p.117.

160. Matthews, *Dissidents: Irish Republican Women, 1923–1941*, pp.84–8.

161. Ibid., p.90.

162. Ibid., p.92.

163. Ibid., p.96.

164. Ibid., pp.100–4.

165. *Irish Nation (Éire),* 5 August 1923.

166. Anonymous, 'Irish Division', *Journal of Mental Science*, 63, 263 (1917), p.620.

167. B. Kelly, 'Female pioneers', *Irish Medical News*, 27 April 2009.

168. D. MacHale and A. Mac Lellan. 'The fabulous Boole sisters', in M. Mulvihill (ed.), *Lab Coats and Lace*, pp.61–71.

169. M. Brück. 'Torch-bearing women astronomers', in M. Mulvihill (ed.), *Lab Coats and Lace*, pp.73–85.

170. C. O'Connell. 'First in their field', in M. Mulvihill (ed.), *Lab Coats and Lace*, pp.37–47.

171. P.N. Wyse Jackson. 'Erratics, intrusions and graptolites', in M. Mulvihill (ed.), *Lab Coats and Lace*, pp.49–59.

172. L. Kelly, *Irish Women in Medicine, c.1880s–1920s: Origins, Education and Careers* (Manchester and New York: Manchester University Press, 2012), pp.160–7; B. Kelly. 'Irish women in medicine', *Irish Medical News*, 7 May 2013; *Irish Times*, 18 May 2013.

173. F. Clarke, 'English, Adeline ('Ada')', in J. McGuire and J. Quinn (eds), *Dictionary of Irish Biography: From the Earliest Times to the Year 2002 (Volume 3, D-F)* (Cambridge: Royal Irish Academy and Cambridge University Press, 2009), pp.626–7; Dickson: *Irish Times*, 12 March 1908.

174. *Irish Times*, 3 June 1895

175. L. Kelly, *Irish Women in Medicine, c.1880s–1920s: Origins, Education and Careers* (Manchester and New York: Manchester University Press, 2012), p.165.

176. *Irish Times*, 24 April 1899.

177. *Irish Times*, 12 July 2011.

178. *Irish Times*, 15 July 2011.

179. Ó hÓgartaigh, *Kathleen Lynn: Irishwoman, Patriot, Doctor*, p.71.

180. Ó hÓgartaigh, *Quiet Revolutionaries: Irish Women in Education, Medicine and Sport, 1861–1964*, p.101.

181. Ó hÓgartaigh, *Kathleen Lynn: Irishwoman, Patriot, Doctor*, p.128.

182. *Irish Times*, 24 October 1921.

183. Ibid.

184. Ibid.

185. Ó hÓgartaigh, *Kathleen Lynn: Irishwoman, Patriot, Doctor*, p.77.

186. *Irish Independent,* 2 June 1919.

187. Matthews, *Renegades*, pp.207–22.

188. *Official Report of the Dáil*, 4 January 1922; *Irish Times*, 5 January 1922.

189. E. Fuller Torrey and J. Miller, *The Invisible Plague: The Rise of Mental Illness from 1750 to the Present* (New Brunswick, NJ and London: Rutgers University Press, 2001), p.154; O. Walsh, 'Gender and insanity in nineteenth-century Ireland', *Clio Medica / The Wellcome Series in the History of Medicine*, 73, 1 (January 2004), pp.69–93; B.D. Kelly, 'Mental health law in Ireland, 1821 to 1902: building the asylums', *Medico-Legal Journal*, 76, 1 (March 2008), pp.19–25; B.D. Kelly, 'Mental health law in Ireland, 1821 to 1902: dealing with the "increase of insanity in Ireland"', *Medico-Legal Journal*, 76, 1 (March 2008), pp.26–33.

190. Healy, *150 Years of British Psychiatry*, pp.268–91.

191. O'Neill, *Irish Mental Health Law*, p.19.

192. E. Boyd Barrett, 'Modern psycho-therapy and our asylums', *Studies*, 13, 49 (March 1924), pp. 9–43; p. 29.

193. Ibid.

194. O'Neill, *Irish Mental Health Law*, p.20.

195. B.D. Kelly, 'The Mental Treatment Act 1945 in Ireland: an historical enquiry', *History of Psychiatry*, 19, 1 (2008), pp.47–67.

196. Quoted in: S.M. Macleod and H.N. McCullough, 'Social science education as a component of medical training', *Social Science and Medicine*, 39, 9 (November 1994), pp.1367–1373.

CHAPTER FIVE

———— ℰᴏ ℭℛ ————

Conclusion: The Legacy of Dr Ada English

On 27 January 1944, English died 'at the Private Nursing Home, Portiuncula, Mount Pleasant, Ballinasloe'.[1] She died of 'coronary thrombosis', a result of heart disease.[2] English's death notice appeared in the *Irish Times*, in both Irish and English, two days after her death:

> English – January 27, 1944, at Ballinasloe, Dr Ada English, RMS, Mental Hospital, Ballinasloe, younger daughter of the late P.J. English and Mrs Nora English, Mullingar. RIP. Remains were taken to St Michael's Church, Ballinasloe yesterday (Friday) evening. Solemn Requiem Mass at 11am (ST) to-day (Saturday) in St Michael's Church. Funeral immediately afterwards to Creagh Cemetry.[3]

English was, 'by her own wish, expressed often ... buried beside some of her old patients in Creagh Cemetery, adjoining the Mental Hospital' in Ballinasloe.[4] Her epitaph reads: 'I ndíl–chuimne ar an Dr Eithne Inglis, Dr Ada English, RMS Mental Hospital Ballinasloe, ball de Cumann na mBan, teachta den dara Dáil, a d'eag ar an 27 Eanar 1944. Go ndéantar do thoil, a Dhia.'[5]

In the *Irish Times*, English's relatives publicly expressed their 'sincere and heartfelt thanks to all those who sympathised' and 'called, sent messages of sympathy, Mass cards and flowers, and to those who attended the funeral and the removal of remains to the church'.[6]

English died without leaving a will. On 17 July 1944 the High Court appointed her brother, Patrick (of Blackrock, Dublin), to administer her personal estate.[7] Her estate was valued at £2,727, eighteen shillings and seven pence.[8] This included a house on Church Street, Ballinasloe valued at £280 and yielding £26 rent annually. At the time of her death, English had £364, nineteen shillings and eight pence in the Ballinasloe branch of the Munster and Leinster Bank and owned Savings Certificates worth £365, seventeen shillings and six pence.

According to J. & E. Davy Stockbrokers of Dublin, English held a total of £1,073, seven shillings and six pence in securities, including Dublin Corporation 5 per cent Inscribed Stock worth £498, seven shillings and six pence, and £20 of shares in Radio Corporation of America, valued at £47. She also held £50 of ordinary stock in Arthur Guinness, Son and Company Limited, valued at £318 and fifteen shillings at the time of her death.

In addition, English jointly held a £1,000 3.25 per cent National Security Loan with her brother Patrick (valued at £1,060) and £70 in 4 per cent preferential stocks in the Great Southern Railway with the 'Reverend John Blowick, Maynooth Mission to China, St Columbans, Navan' (valued at £34 and thirteen shillings). English had been receiving income on both holdings up to her death and, according to the *Schedule of Assets*, both were purchased 'with the intention that they should pass to the other joint holder on her death'.[9] Finally, English had, throughout her career, contributed £471, eight shillings and eleven pence to the Superannuation Fund at the hospital in Ballinasloe.

Following her death, English's personal effects were auctioned by John Cunningham, auctioneer, valuer and general merchant from Main Street, Ballinasloe. They raised the total sum of £259, four shillings and nine pence. In addition, she left a clock in a case (valued at £2 and ten shillings), an R.G. Cushion watch (£2) and a silver cigarette case (fifteen shillings), which were valued into her estate.

The ultimate fate of English's personal effects is unknown. Nor is it known what personal papers, letters or diaries she may have left, or what became of them. As a result, any examination of English's legacy must focus chiefly on the public record of her life and contributions to medicine and politics.

Political Legacy

English was highly active in Irish political life during a uniquely eventful time in modern Ireland. She was an active member of the Irish Volunteers and Cumann na mBan, participated in the War of Independence, and, in 1921, spent several months in Galway jail, for possessing nationalist literature. While in jail, English was elected to the Second Dáil where she spoke strongly against the Anglo-Irish Treaty. She was involved in the Civil War and was linked with 'Miss MacSwiney's Dáil' in January 1929.[10] In addition, English's strong nationalist outlook was apparent throughout all other aspects of her life, including her work at Ballinasloe District Asylum.[11] Despite these involvements, English is not commonly remembered as a major political figure.

This situation is regrettable and is likely attributable to the fact that English's contributions to these events are less well-documented than her contributions to mental healthcare, despite the fact that she participated in key phases of the struggle for Irish independence. In political terms, English was not a major leader within the republican movement and nor was she one of the defining political personalities of the era. But neither was she a minor participant: her time in prison in Galway and election to the Second Dáil indicate the depth of her commitment to the cause of Irish independence. Her contribution was, then, both considerable and considered, and her dedication to the struggle was unwavering.

In terms of her background, English had much in common not only with fellow-republican doctors like Lynn, Price, Thornton and Fleury, but also with many other participants in movements such as Cumann na mBan and the Irish Suffrage Movement, many of whom were, like English, Roman Catholic, nationalist, upper-middle class women.[12] The personal political contributions of some of these women are remembered individually, but many are not.

Up until 2011, the sole public commemoration of English's political contribution was an annual commemoration by Sinn Féin in Ballinasloe. In 2011, however, English's political contributions emerged as a key theme at the inaugural Ada English Summer School in Ballinasloe.[13]

This commemorative event was organised by the Association of Irish Festival Events and the Ballinasloe and District Branch of Soroptomists International, a worldwide service organisation for women, committed to a world where women and girls together achieve their potential, realise aspirations and have an equal voice in creating strong, peaceful communities. The Symposium involved a range of participants including historians, academics, gender studies specialists and doctors discussing English's life and legacy. There were lectures, debates, entertainments and a walking tour of the grounds of St Brigid's Hospital, Ballinasloe, with an especially poignant pause at the RMS's house on the grounds of the hospital, where English had lived. Attendees also visited English's grave, across the road in Creagh Cemetry, where a wreath was laid.

In its second year (2012), the Ada English Symposium featured an even broader range of events including an exhibition of memorabilia from St Brigid's Hospital and a lively discussion on women in politics, articulating strongly the political legacy of English and other early women members of the Houses of Oireachtas.[14] The third year (2013) saw continued expansion with lectures on medicine and the asylum, the economic impact of St Brigid's Hospital, schizophrenia in the late nineteenth and early twentieth centuries, children's burial grounds, and the Earls of Clancarty, local land owners.[15] There was a symposium about St Brigid's Hospital, a presentation of art work by Úna Spain, and wreath-laying at English's grave. Relatives of English presented the inaugural Ada English Trophy for camogie, a sport that English promoted strongly during her time in Ballinasloe.[16]

These symposia are fitting tributes to an individual whose life combined politics and medicine with a strong social conscience, and showed a profound commitment to reformist and revolutionary activism in both spheres. Ultimately, English's deepest connection was with her patients in Ballinasloe, to whom she devoted almost four decades of her life: it is fitting she is remembered there.

Medical Legacy

From a medical perspective, English was one of the first generation of female medical graduates in Ireland and Great Britain, graduating as a doctor from the Royal University, Dublin in 1903. She spent almost four decades working at Ballinasloe Mental Hospital during a particularly difficult era in the history of Irish mental health services, characterised by large custodial institutions, which were often over-crowded and poorly therapeutic. During her time in Ballinasloe, English oversaw several significant innovations, including improvements in patients' living conditions, the development and expansion of occupational therapy programmes, and early introduction of convulsive treatment for severe mental illness.

However, Irish mental hospitals remained in a regrettable state for much of the first half of the twentieth century. In 1924, in the midst of English's time in Ballinasloe, Edward Boyd Barrett SJ drew attention to the asylums, noting that there was 'practically no treatment'[17] and calling for 'scientific treatment of curable cases'.[18] The introduction of Cardiazol convulsive treatment at the Ballinasloe Asylum in 1939 represents one of the most historically significant therapeutic developments during English's time working there and, indeed, in the history of Irish psychiatry in the early twentieth century. Further research is needed into the broader history of convulsive treatment in Ireland, but, at present, this reference to Cardiazol treatment by Committee of Management in Ballinasloe in 1939 is the earliest known reference to convulsive treatment in an Irish context.

One of the other treatments to emerge during this period was occupational therapy and, as the *Irish Times* noted in her obituary, English 'developed occupational therapy to a high degree' at Ballinasloe.[19] English was by no means alone in her promotion of occupational therapy in Irish asylums; others, such as Dr Eamonn O'Sullivan in Killarney Mental Hospital[20] were working along similar lines.[21] Nonetheless, in 1939 the 'occupational therapy department' in Ballinasloe drew the particular attention of the Inspector of Mental Hospitals, who noted that 'a total of 996 patients are engaged in various occupations, as many as 250 being employed on the farm; others are engaged at various trades and handicrafts ... the amusements – both indoor and outdoor – of the patients are well catered for; dances are held weekly during the winter months'.[22]

In Ballinasloe, the emphasis on novel treatments for mental illness, occupational therapy and other measures to improve the lives of patients (sports, cinema trips, etc.) was attributable, in large part, to the tireless work and advocacy of English. These initiatives reflect a broad-based, socially-minded approach to health and wellbeing which was also apparent in English's contribution to the Irish Catholic Truth Society Conference in 1921, when she advocated for 'decent housing for the working classes for it was impossible that people who were condemned to dwell in wretched, crowded insanitary houses could cherish or practice any high ideals either of religion or nationality'.[23]

On that occasion, English also stated that there 'were social and national movements which necessarily drew people from the home life, and they should be prepared to take their share in these movements'.[24] In her own life, English played a considerable role in such 'movements', especially the nationalist movement, alongside her busy medical career. To this extent, English's life and work showed significant similarities with those of Lynn, Lyons and Fleury, another asylum doctor (see Chapter Four).

English belongs firmly within this group of politically active, socially-minded doctors, combining strong political views with progressive medical practice, underpinned by a clear focus on improving health-care for children, the poor, the disadvantaged and, in the case of English and Fleury, the forgotten patients of Ireland's vast asylum system. Together, these individuals made substantial contributions to the emerging Irish state in dramatic, memorable ways (participating in republican movements and uprisings, being repeatedly imprisoned) but also in quieter, arguably more profound ways (reforming health care, advocating for the poor).

From a medical perspective, English focused her medical work on an especially intractable problem: Ireland's monolithic asylum system. The task of reforming Ireland's asylum system was an enormous and important one, and one which was, inevitably, unfinished at the time of English's death.

Reforming Mental Health Services in Twentieth-Century Ireland

The overall quality and level of mental health service provision continued to give cause for concern well into the 1940s. In 1944, the anonymous psychiatrist, writing in *The Bell*, noted that despite improvements in facilities for the mentally ill in 'neighbouring countries', the 'Irish Government lagged behind and, even though many years have passed, that lag is still apparent'.[25]

Consistent with the report of the *Commission on the Relief of the Sick and Destitute Poor, including Insane Poor,*[26] the anonymous psychiatrist lamented the absence of a voluntary admission status in Irish asylums, but added that 'it is not too much to hope that legislation in the near future will remedy this and provide for the admission of voluntary patients'.[27] A voluntary admission process was indeed introduced the following year, as part of the Mental Treatment Act 1945, an innovative piece of legislation that introduced many important reforms to Irish mental health services[28] and was to remain in force until the Mental Health Act 2001 was fully implemented in 2006.[29]

English had, however, died in 1944, one year prior to the long-awaited Mental Treatment Act 1945. There can be little doubt that English would have welcomed many of the reforms in the 1945 Act, especially the simplification of admission processes and the aspiration towards more accessible, less custodial services for the mentally ill. In August 1939, when English was Acting RMS, the Committee of Management at Ballinasloe had issued a strong resolution 'calling for a revision of the existing lunacy laws dealing with both the reception and after treatment of mental cases'.[30]

When the revised law was finally passing through Seanad Éireann (the upper house of the Irish parliament) on 19 April 1945, Mrs Helena Concannon, an historian and Senator for the National University of Ireland constituency, paid tribute to English's dedication to improving conditions for the mentally ill:

> One melancholy note resounded in my heart when I read in the newspapers last November the report of the Second Reading in the Dáil of the measure we are now considering. It was that the late Dr Ada English had not been spared to be present when the Parliamentary Secretary was introducing it. He knows – because he, too, had the privilege of knowing well that great-hearted woman – all that I have in mind when I speak thus. All her life, since she entered the mental hospital service as a brilliant and beautiful girl until she was laid to rest, as she herself desired, in the little God's Acre near Ballinasloe, where many of her poor patients await the Resurrection – she worked for the principles embodied in this Bill. The things that make it memorable and worthwhile are things for which she tirelessly pleaded. Some of them were accepted, in principle at least, when in 1925 the term 'mental hospital' replaced the old, depressing designation of 'lunatic asylum'. Implicit in the new designation was the acceptance of the thesis that mental disease is not a crime, but a disease, like any other disease, capable

of being cured if proper curative measures can be applied in time. A mental hospital is, therefore, first of all, a place for such curative treatment and not merely a place of detention for unfortunates thus afflicted. She always felt that conditions should be such that the physicians in charge should not be so overburdened with administrative detail that they could not spare the time needed for their own proper job – time to study their patients and to give them the undivided care their condition calls for. Another necessity she tirelessly stressed was that of establishing mental clinics, such as are contemplated in the Bill, where incipient mental disorders might be detected, and their progress stayed by expert treatment to which patients might voluntarily submit themselves. This aim is recognised, too, in important provisions of the present Bill.[31]

As this moving tribute demonstrates, English, 'a brilliant and beautiful girl', played an important role in efforts to reform and renew Irish mental health services throughout the 1920s, 1930s and 1940s, and made a particular contribution to the improvement of conditions in Ballinalsoe. As the *Irish Times* noted, English truly 'did a great deal to bring about the changes which transferred the lunatic asylum into the present mental hospital'.[32] Despite English's work, however, there was still much to be done.

In 1924, Boyd Barrett had outlined his vision of a reformed asylum system which would facilitate the 'scientific treatment of curable cases' and be complemented by 'nerve clinics … where advice and treatment should be available for ordinary cases of nerve trouble and incipient insanity'.[33] Although progress had been made on achieving this vision during the course of English's career, the process of reform was by no means complete by the time she retired in 1942. Indeed, some seventy years after English's retirement there remained elements of Boyd Barrett's vision that had not been fulfilled, as the Inspector of Mental Health Services in 2012 lamented a recent 'catastrophic reduction in staffing numbers'[34] and the fact 'that staff re-deployment has taken place from the community to inpatient units and staff, formerly allocated to therapeutic activities, have been transferred to duties more custodial in nature'.[35] The Inspector also expressed concern about a range of other, more specific matters, including that fact that there was 'no specific unit providing for the acute treatment of intellectually disabled people with serious mental health problems'.[36]

Despite these persistent deficits, a certain amount of progress was made during English's working life, as evidenced by the account provided in 1944, two years after English retired, by the anonymous psychiatrist in *The Bell*. This psychiatrist admitted that 'the change has been a gradual one' but, finally, 'the gaoler with the whip was replaced by the doctor', and then 'the old-fashioned doctor with his copious blood-letting' was replaced by 'the specialist'.[37] Even so, there was clear room for further improvement:

> To-day [1943/4] the treatment of mental disease is in its infancy and it is no wild hope to say that the mental experts of 2000 AD will write of 'the crude, unscientific treatment of mental disease in 1943'.[38]

The anonymous psychiatrist had specific advice for those, like English, who sought to reform Ireland's asylum system:

> The tendency everywhere is to laud the genius, but it is by the average man and woman that the world is run and saved from being a worse world. If psychology has a great lesson for the average citizen – that of accepting necessary restrictions – it has also a very important one for the governors and reformers: for the one – *Do not restrict more than is necessary*; and for the other – *Hasten slowly*.[39]

English was just such a steady, dogged reformer throughout her career in Ballinasloe, seeking to improve conditions for patients at local level as well as advocating reform at national level. Her dedication to her Ballinasloe patients was absolute and, as she had often requested, English was finally buried alongside them in Creagh Cemetery, where her grave still lies within sight of her beloved St Brigid's Hospital.[40]

Conclusion

On 27 January 1945, one year after English's death, a short commemorative notice appeared in the *Irish Times*: 'Inglis – I ndíl-chuimhne ar an Dr Eithne Inglis (Dr Ada English, Ballinasloe), a d'éag an 27ú Mí d'Eanair, 1944. "For a little lonely while." Beannacht leat.'[41] The closing quotation in this moving notice is taken from a poem titled *Beannacht Leat*, written by Ethna Carbery:

> *Beannacht leat!*
> I hold your hand in mine, I say
> The parting words this parting day –
> And if a sob be stifled, Dear,
> I pray you turn aside, nor hear –
> I would be brave, and yet, and yet,
> Can we two sunder without regret?

Beannacht leat!
May every vagrant wind a-stir
Between us be a messenger,
Each falling wild-rose petal blow
A haunting perfume where you go,
And all the brown birds in the blue
Sing memories of me to you.

Beannacht leat!
Thank God! 'tis not a long good-bye
We give each other, you and I –
Sure in my heart the hope is fain
To whisper, You will come again
With the kind eyes, the same kind smile –
Then for a little lonely while,
Beannacht leat![42]

Carbery, who wrote the poem, was an Irish journalist, poet and publisher best known for writing the ballad *Rody McCorley*. She was a member of Inghinidhe na hÉireann (Daughters of Ireland), a radical Irish nationalist women's organisation led by Maud Gonne, which later merged with Cumann na mBan, of which English was a member.[43] Clearly, English and Carbery found common ground in their commitment to Irish nationalism, and it is fitting that Carbery's words were used publicly to commemorate English following her death.

Today, English is chiefly remembered as an 'extraordinary lady psychiatrist'[44] who, as Senator Mary Henry notes, 'worked tirelessly ... because of her devotion to her Ballinasloe patients'.[45] In this way, English made a unique contribution to the development of public mental health services at a time when reform was very badly needed, not least through her ultimately successful advocacy for improved mental health legislation.

It is also true, however, that English's vision extended well beyond the asylum walls, so that 'the plight of the poor and the care of mentally ill patients became her twin children'.[46] With this in mind, English was continually engaged, in the broadest possible way, in efforts to build an Irish state that was equitable, just and, most of all, free.[47]

This was, perhaps, English's most revolutionary contribution of all: seeking to build better services for the mentally ill *and* fight for social justice and freedom for all, especially those who were marginalised, forgotten and downtrodden.

And there are still none more marginalised and forgotten than those to whom English devoted her life's work: the mentally ill, who are still commonly constrained to live lives characterised by stigma, social exclusion and denial of human rights.[48] English's work is, as yet, unfinished.

Notes

1. *East Galway Democrat*, 29 January 1944; *Irish Press*, 28 January 1944.
2. Adeline English, Death Certificate (General Register Office/An tSeirbhís um Chlárú Sibhialta, Roscommon, Ireland).
3. *Irish Times*, 29 January 1944.
4. *Irish Press*, 28 January 1944; *East Galway Democrat*, 29 January 1944. See also: F. Clarke, 'English, Adeline ('Ada')', in J. McGuire and J. Quinn (eds), *Dictionary of Irish Biography: From the Earliest Times to the Year 2002 (Volume 3, D-F)* (Cambridge: Royal Irish Academy and Cambridge University Press, 2009), pp.626–7.
5. 'In beloved memory of Dr Ada English, RMS Mental Hospital Ballinasloe, member of Cumann na mBan, member of the Second Dáil, who died on 27 January 1944. May thy will be done, God.'
6. *Irish Times*, 12 February 1944.
7. Grant of Administration (Adeline English) 17 July 1944 (National Archives, Bishop Street, Dublin, Ireland).
8. Schedule of Assets (Adeline English) 17 July 1944 (National Archives, Bishop Street, Dublin, Ireland) (signed by English's brother, Patrick Francis English, 8 June 1944).
9. Ibid.
10. *Irish Times*, 22 January 1929.
11. M. Davoren, E.G. Breen and B.D. Kelly, 'Dr Adeline English: revolutionizing politics and psychiatry in Ireland', *Irish Psychiatrist*, 10, 4 (Winter 2009), pp.260–2.
12. Ferriter, *The Transformation of Ireland 1900–2000*, p.176.
13. R. Moore, 'Inaugural Ada English Symposium planned', *Ballinasloe Life*, 1 (2011), p.29.
14. A. O'Connor, 'Forget gender quotas, we need more Brigids in Dáil', *Irish Independent*, 12 May 2012.
15. O. Dunne, '3rd Ada English Summer School', *Ballinasloe Life*, 3, 1 (April/May 2013), p.34.
16. Mac Loughlin, *Ballinasloe Inniú agus Inné*, p.144.
17. E. Boyd Barrett, 'Modern psycho-therapy and our asylums', *Studies*, 13, 49 (March 1924), pp.9–43.
18. Boyd Barrett, 'Modern psycho-therapy and our asylums', p.43.
19. *Irish Times*, 29 January 1944.
20. Fogarty, *Dr Eamonn O'Sullivan*.
21. O'Sullivan, *Textbook of Occupational Therapy*.
22. Minutes of the Proceedings of the Committee of Management of Ballinasloe District Asylum, 8 April 1940.
23. *Irish Times*, 24 October 1921.
24. Ibid.
25. Psychiatrist, 'Insanity in Ireland', *The Bell*, 7, 4 (January 1944), pp.303–10.

26. O'Neill, *Irish Mental Health Law*.
27. Psychiatrist, 'Insanity in Ireland', *The Bell*, 7, 4 (January 1944), pp.303–10.
28. B.D. Kelly, 'The Mental Treatment Act 1945 in Ireland: an historical enquiry', *History of Psychiatry*, 19, 1 (March 2008), pp.47–67. See also: *Irish Times*, 10 March 1959.
29. B.D. Kelly, 'Ireland's Mental Health Act 2001', *Psychiatric Bulletin*, 31, 1 (January 2007), pp.21–4.
30. Minutes of the Proceedings of the Committee of Management of Ballinasloe District Asylum, 14 August 1939.
31. Official Report of Seanad Éireann (Houses of Oireachtas, Dublin, Ireland) (Vol. 29 No. 25), 19 April 1945.
32. *Irish Times*, 29 January 1944.
33. Boyd Barrett, 'Modern psycho-therapy and our asylums', p.43.
34. Inspector of Mental Health Services, *Report of the Inspector of Mental Health Services 2011* (Dublin: Mental Health Commission, 2012), p.75.
35. Inspector of Mental Health Services, *Report of the Inspector of Mental Health Services 2011*, p.77.
36. Inspector of Mental Health Services, *Report of the Inspector of Mental Health Services 2011*, p.80. This is a long-standing problem in Irish mental health services. See: B.D. Kelly, 'One hundred years ago: the Richmond Asylum, Dublin in 1907', *Irish Journal of Psychological Medicine*, 24, 3 (2007), pp.108–14; B.D. Kelly, 'Learning disability and forensic mental healthcare in nineteenth-century Ireland', *Irish Journal of Psychological Medicine*, 25, 3 (2008), pp.116–18; B.D. Kelly, 'Intellectual disability, mental illness and offending behaviour: forensic cases from early twentieth century Ireland', *Irish Journal of Medical Science*, 179, 3 (2010), pp.409–16.
37. Psychiatrist, 'Insanity in Ireland', *The Bell*, 7, 4 (January 1944), p.305.
38. Ibid.
39. Ibid., p.310.
40. McNamara and Mooney, *Women in Parliament: 1918–2000*, p.79.
41. *Irish Times*, 27 January 1945: 'English – In beloved memory of Dr Adeline English (Dr Ada English, Ballinasloe), who died on the 27 January 1944. "For a little lonely while." Blessings be with you.'
42. E. Carbery, *The Four Winds of Eirinn: Poems by Ethna Carbery (Anna MacManus) Complete Edition*, (Dublin: M. H. Gill and Son, 1906), p.136. 'Beannacht leat' means 'Blessings be with you' (in Irish).
43. Kelly, *Between the Lines of History*, p.25; McNamara and Mooney, *Women in Parliament*, p.79; M. Clancy, 'On the "Western Outpost": Local government and women's suffrage in county Galway', in G. Moran (ed.), *Galway: History and Society – Interdisciplinary Essays on the History of an Irish County* (Dublin: Geography Publications, 1996), pp.557–87; p.562; Witness Statement (Number 568) of Eilis, Bean Uí Chonaill (Dublin: Bureau of Military History, 1913–21, File Number S.1846), p.55; Witness Statement (Number 1,752) of Mrs McCarvill (Eileen McGrane) (Dublin: Bureau of Military History, 1913–21, File Number S.1434), p.7; *Irish Press*, 28 January 1944; *East Galway Democrat*, 29 January 1944.
44. M. Gueret, 'A lovely idea', *Sunday Independent*, 17 July 2011. See also: E. Fitzgerald, 'There's women for you', *Irish Times*, 16 December 2000.

45. M. Henry, 'Medical women in parliament', *Irish Medical News*, 30 January 2001.
46. M. Gueret, 'A lovely idea', *Sunday Independent*, 17 July 2011.
47. B.D. Kelly, 'Dr Ada English (1875–1944); doctor, patriot, politician', *British Journal of Psychiatry*, 204, 1 (January 2014), p.5.
48. B.D. Kelly, 'Structural violence and schizophrenia', *Social Science and Medicine*, 61, 3 (2005), pp.721–30; B.D. Kelly, 'The power gap: freedom, power and mental illness', *Social Science and Medicine*, 63, 8 (2006), pp.2118–28; B.D. Kelly, 'Mental illness and structural violence', *Irish Medical Journal*, 105, 1 (2012), p.30.

— ℰ ℛ —

Chronology of the Life and Times of Dr Adeline (Ada) English (1875–1944)

Year	Historical Events	Events in the Life of Dr Adeline (Ada) English
1800–01	The Acts of Union unite the Kingdom of Great Britain and Kingdom of Ireland to create the United Kingdom of Great Britain and Ireland. Ireland remains part of the United Kingdom of Great Britain and Ireland until 6 December 1922 when the Irish Free State comes into being.	
1833	Connaught District Lunatic Asylum opens in Ballinasloe at a cost of £27,000, with capacity for 150 patients.	

Year	Historical Events	Events in the Life of Dr Adeline (Ada) English
1841	The Association of Medical Officers of Asylums for the Insane is founded by Dr Samuel Hitch in England. It later changes its name to the Medico-Psychological Association (1864).	
1845–52	The Great Irish Famine occurs, resulting in one million deaths and one million people emigrating.	
1867	Dr Eleonora Fleury is born; she later becomes the first medical graduate of the Royal University of Ireland (1890) and first female member of the Medico-Psychological Association (1894); she works at the Richmond and Portrane Asylums (Dublin) and is imprisoned for hiding and treating republican fugitives in the asylums (1923).	
1874	Dr Kathleen Lynn is born; she later co-founds St Ultan's Hospital for Infants, with Madeleine ffrench-Mullen, in Dublin (1919) and is a Sinn Féin member of the Fourth Dáil (1923-27).	
1875		10 January. English is born in Caherciveen, County Kerry, to Nora (Mulvihill) and Patrick English.

Year	Historical Events	Events in the Life of Dr Adeline (Ada) English
1876	The Medical Qualifications Act removes the legal restriction on women entering the profession of medicine.	
1878	The Intermediate Education Act is passed in Ireland, giving girls access to all examinations of the Intermediate Board.	
1879	The Land League is founded in County Mayo, to fight for the 'three Fs': fair rent, fixity of tenure and free sale. The 'Land War' follows (1880–82).	English, growing up in Mullingar, is aware of the suffering of the poor as her grandfather is master of the nearby Oldcastle Workhouse, County Meath.
1881		The Loreto Convent is established in Mullingar, County Westmeath on a site donated by Lord Greville, member of parliament for Westmeath (1865–74); English attends school there.
1885	The Medical School of the Royal College of Surgeons in Ireland became the first medical school in Great Britain and Ireland to admit women to its lectures.	
1890	Dr Dorothy Price (1890–1954) is born; she later serves as medical officer to a Cork brigade of the Irish Republican Army and plays a key role in the eradication of tuberculosis in Ireland.	

Year	Historical Events	Events in the Life of Dr Adeline (Ada) English
1898	Dr Brigid Lyons Thornton (1898–1987) is born; she later works with Michael Collins (1890–1922) during the War of Independence; works in public health; and becomes librarian at the Rotunda Hospital in Dublin.	
1899		English attends Irish classes at the Jesuit University College, Dublin, given by Pádraig Pearse (1879–1916); James Joyce (1882–1941) also attends.
1903	A Conference of the Irish Asylums Committee at the Richmond Hospital in Dublin seeks solutions to the inexorable rise in demand for asylum beds in Ireland.	English graduates from the Catholic University School of Medicine (MB BS). *St Stephen's*, college magazine of the Catholic University, congratulates English on her examination results.
1904	Irish asylums are significantly over-crowded, with 1293 patients in Ballinasloe District Asylum (774 male, 519 female); of these, 311 are 'under treatment' (203 male, 108 female).	English registers as a medical doctor (16 February). English gains experience at the Mater Misericordiae Hospital, Richmond Asylum and Children's Hospital, Temple Street, Dublin. English is appointed 'second assistant medical officer' in Ballinasloe District Asylum (12 September).

Year	Historical Events	Events in the Life of Dr Adeline (Ada) English
1905	Sinn Féin is established (28 November) by Arthur Griffith (1872–1922), an Irish writer, politician and, later, President of Dáil Éireann (10 January to 12 August 1922).	In Ballinasloe District Asylum, English and her colleague, Dr Richard Kirwan, have the Galway Arms emblazoned place of Queen Victoria on the buttons of uniforms; promote Irish-manufactured products; and are involved in the Ballinasloe branch of Conradh na Gaeilge (Gaelic League)
1910		English and Kirwan are active in the establishment of Sinn Féin in Ballinasloe.
1913	The Irish Volunteers is founded (25 November).	English applies (unsuccessfully) for the post of 'Tuberculosis Officer for Roscommon', reflecting the problems presented by tuberculosis in asylums.
1914	Cumann na mBan is founded (2 April). A bill introducing 'home rule' for Ireland (the Government of Ireland Act) is passed but does not come into effect owing to World War I and the Easter Rising.	English continues to work in Ballinasloe District Asylum where particular emphasis is placed on sport: the asylum team makes the final of the St Grellan League and English (a keen golfer) is largely responsible for the introduction of camogie; the hospital camogie team duly becomes one of the best in the country.
1914–18	World War I	English organises Red Cross lectures in Ballinasloe during World War I.

Year	Historical Events	Events in the Life of Dr Adeline (Ada) English
1916	The Easter Rising takes place (24–29 April) and an Irish Republic is proclaimed at the General Post Office in Dublin (24 April).	English reportedly serves as medical officer for rebels in County Galway, under the command of Liam Mellows (1895–1922).
	Fifteen of the leaders of the Rising, including Pádraig Pearse (1879–1916, a friend of English), are executed.	The Lunacy Inspectors tell the Committee of Management of Ballinasloe District Asylum of 'scandalous' conditions in parts of the asylum; English, as acting Resident Medical Superintendent (RMS) agrees immediate action is needed.
		The Committee of Management 'determinedly protest[s] against the exclusion of any portion of Ulster from the scheme of national government … the division of Ireland we will not have' (12 June).
		English withdraws her application for the post of RMS and Dr John Mills is elected (9 October).
1916		The Summer Meeting of the Irish Division of the Medico-Psychological Association is held in Ballinasloe at the invitation of Dr Mills (July); English attends.
		Dr John Dignan (1880–1953), friend of English and later Bishop of the Diocese of Clonfert (1924–53), is elected president of the East Galway branch of Sinn Féin.

Year	Historical Events	Events in the Life of Dr Adeline (Ada) English
1914–43	English's *alma mater*, the Catholic University School of Medicine at Cecilia Street closes in 1931 without ever appointing a woman to its academic staff.	English is lecturer and examiner in 'mental diseases' at Queen's College, Galway.
1918	Sinn Féin is successful in the Irish elections, winning seventy-three of Ireland's 105 seats in the British House of Commons. Constance Markievicz (1868–1927) becomes the first woman elected to the British House of Commons. Sinn Féin members do not take up their seats.	English is local president of Cumann na mBan in Ballinasloe and a member of Sinn Féin in Galway; she actively demonstrates against conscription in Ballinasloe.
1919	Dáil Éireann (the First Dáil) is declared in Dublin (21 January) and Éamon de Valera (1882–1975) is elected President of Dáil Éireann (1 April 1919 to 26 August 1921). An 'asylum soviet' is established in Monaghan in the context of industrial unrest in Irish asylums.	
1919–21	The War of Independence with Great Britain occurs. George Clancy (1881–1921) (republican mayor of Limerick and friend of English) is shot by British forces.	English is an executive member of Cumann na mBan and the delegate from County Galway to the Annual Convention of Cumann na mBan (1919–20).

Year	Historical Events	Events in the Life of Dr Adeline (Ada) English
	A truce is struck on 11 July 1921.	English uses job offers at the asylum in Ballinasloe to help persuade members of the Royal Irish Constabulary to leave the organisation.
		English is arrested (19 January 1921); sentenced to nine months in Galway jail for illegal possession of documents (24 February); and released early owing to food poisoning (13 May).
		English speaks at the Catholic Truth Society in Dublin, emphasising the necessity for citizens to take part in 'social and national movements', and the importance of 'decent housing for the working classes' if they are to 'cherish and practice any high ideals wither of religion or nationality' (23 October).
1921	Following elections, the Second Dáil convenes (16 August 1921 to 8 June 1922). Éamon de Valera is elected President of the Irish Republic (26 August 1921 to 9 January 1922).	The Committee of Management of Ballinasloe District Asylum resolves that 'henceforth no communication of any kind be forwarded to any department of the British Government in Ireland' (11 July).
		Austin Stack offers English promotion to the position of RMS of Sligo Mental Hospital; she refuses to be separated from her patients in Ballinasloe.

Year	Historical Events	Events in the Life of Dr Adeline (Ada) English
		English is one of six Sinn Féin women elected to the Second Dáil; she is an unopposed Sinn Féin candidate for the National University of Ireland Constituency (16 August).
		English speaks in Dáil Éireann in strong support of the nomination of Éamon de Valera as President of the Irish Republic (26 August).
1921–2	The Anglo-Irish Treaty is signed (6 December 1921).	English speaks in Dáil Éireann in strong opposition to the Treaty (4 January 1922) which is nonetheless ratified by Dáil Éireann (sixty-four members in favour, fifty-seven against, including English) (7 January).
1922	Elections are held for the Third Dáil and pro-Treaty Sinn Féin (led by Michael Collins) win fifty-eight out of 128 seats while anti-Treaty Sinn Féin (led by Éamon de Valera) win thirty-six.	English, an anti-Treaty candidate, is not re-elected; her seat is taken by Professor William Magennis, an independent candidate.
1922–3	The Civil War occurs. Liam Mellows (anti-Treaty republican and friend of English) is executed by Free State (pro-Treaty) forces (8 December 1922). Michael Collins (pro-Treaty leader) is killed in an ambush at Béal na mBláth in County Cork (22 August 1922).	English (anti-Treaty) is in Dublin during the occupation of the Four Courts by anti-Treaty members of the Irish Republican Army (April 1922). English reportedly serves with Cathal Brugha (1874–1922) at the Hammam Hotel on Sackville Street (later O'Connell Street) in Dublin (June 1922).

Year	Historical Events	Events in the Life of Dr Adeline (Ada) English
	Liam Lynch (anti–Treaty leader) is killed in an ambush in County Tipperary (10 April 1923). A ceasefire is declared (24 May 1923).	Brugha is killed (7 July 1922). English is arrested by the (pro–Treaty) Provisional Government (August 1922).
1924	An article in *Studies* by Edward Boyd Barrett SJ, bemoans the state of public asylums in Ireland and especially the lack of effective treatments.	Ongoing industrial unrest at Ballinasloe District Asylum as staff go on strike and Civic Guards are requisitioned for duty at the hospital; the matter is resolved when the gate porter (non-union) resigns.
1929	'Miss MacSwiney's Dáil', established by Mary MacSwiney (1872–1942) (anti–Treaty republican politician and educationalist), meets at the Rotunda in Dublin (21 January) and does not recognise the legitimacy of the new Dáil.	English is listed as an 'absentee member' of 'Miss MacSwiney's Dáil'. Dr Kathleen Lynn (1874–1955) (republican politician and pioneering doctor) is present.
1932		English is a guest at a State Reception at Dublin Castle, hosted by President de Valera, with Cardinal Bourne, Archbishop of Westminster, and other religious leaders (21 June) on the occasion of the Eucharistic Congress of Dublin (22–26 June).

Year	Historical Events	Events in the Life of Dr Adeline (Ada) English
1936		The Local Appointments Commissioners reject English's application for the post of Resident Medical Superintendent in favour of Dr Bernard Lyons, much to the displeasure of the Committee of Management of Ballinasloe Mental Hospital and Ballinasloe Urban Council.
1939	World War II commences.	The Committee of Management of Ballinasloe District Asylum is informed that 'modern treatments of mental patients' are being tried at the hospital (20 November). The Committee hears that 'that the Minister [for Local Government] has no objection to the proposal to carry out Cardiazol treatment on certain patients provided the RMS accepts responsibility' (11 December); this is the first known reference to convulsive therapy in Ireland. English organises Red Cross lectures in Ballinasloe during World War II.

Year	Historical Events	Events in the Life of Dr Adeline (Ada) English
1940		A sworn enquiry is held at Ballinasloe Mental Hospital (3 to 5 January) with the result that the Committee of Management is dissolved; the RMS (Dr Lyons) becomes medical officer in Castlerea Branch Mental Asylum; the Matron is retired on pension; the Minister confirms that 'English has discharged her duties efficiently'; and English becomes acting RMS (11 June). English reports that the military have taken over part of the asylum, trenches are dug and air-raid shelters provided; English reports that 'the military have been very kind and helpful to us in advice and supervision' (8 July). English arranges for patients to attend the cinema in Ballinasloe town (12 August).
1941		English, aged sixty-six years, is finally appointed RMS after thirty-seven years working in Ballinasloe (10 June).
1942		English submits her letter of resignation to Ballinasloe Mental Hospital (11 August).

Year	Historical Events	Events in the Life of Dr Adeline (Ada) English
1944	An article in *The Bell*, written by an anonymous psychiatrist, argues that mental health services in Ireland lag behind services elsewhere, but that recent decades had finally seen some progress.	English dies of 'coronary thrombosis', a result of heart disease, at Mount Pleasant Nursing Home (later Portiuncula Hospital), Ballinasloe. English leaves an estate valued at £2,727, eighteen shillings and seven pence. English's personal effects are auctioned.
1945	The Mental Treatment Act introduces much-needed reforms to Irish mental health services, including revised procedures for involuntary admission, and voluntary admission status.	English's strong advocacy for the mentally ill is acknowledged in the Senate in a moving tribute by Senator Helena Concannon, who describes English as a 'brilliant and beautiful girl' who 'worked for the principles embodied in this Bill' and says that 'the things that make [this Act] worthwhile are things for which she tirelessly pleaded' (19 April).
1949	The Republic of Ireland comes into being (18 April).	
2011		The inaugural Ada English Summer School takes place in Ballinasloe.

BIBLIOGRAPHY

—————— ℰ ℭ ——————

PRIMARY SOURCES

Manuscripts

Apothecaries' Hall of Ireland Roll of Licentiates (Commencing April 1913) (Royal College of Physicians of Ireland, Dublin, Ireland).

Birth Certificate, Adeline English, 10 January 1875 (General Register Office/ An tSeirbhís um Chlárú Sibhialta, Roscommon, Ireland).

Bureau of Military History 1913–21 Collection Witness Statements (Military Archives, Cathal Brugha Barracks, Dublin):

- Witness Statement (Number 366) of Alice M. Cashel (File Number S.1420).
- Witness Statement (Number 568) of Eilis, Bean Uí Chonaill (File Number S.1846).
- Witness Statement (Number 624) of Mrs Mary Flannery Woods (File Number S.1901).
- Witness Statement (Number 806) of Mrs George Clancy (Máire, Bean Mhic Fhlannachadha) (File Number S.2117).
- Witness Statement (Number 1,062) of Laurence Garvey (File Number S.2367).
- Witness Statement (Number 1,219) of Sean O'Neill (File Number S.2451).
- Witness Statement (Number 1,752) of Mrs McCarvill (Eileen McGrane) (File Number S.1434).

Census Return Forms for House One in Ballybeg (Clareabbey, County Clare), 31 March 1901 (The National Archives of Ireland, Dublin).

Census Return Forms for House Thirteen in Earls South Side (Mullingar Urban, Westmeath), 31 March 1901 (The National Archives of Ireland, Dublin).

Census Return Forms for House Eight in Earl Street (Mullingar South Urban, Westmeath), 2 April 1911 (The National Archives of Ireland, Dublin).

Census Return Forms for House Ninety-Eight in Burrow South (Howth, County Dublin), 2 April 1911 (The National Archives of Ireland, Dublin).

Death Certificate, Adeline English, 21 March 1944 (General Register Office/ An tSeirbhís um Chlárú Sibhialta, Roscommon, Ireland).

General Register of Prisoners, Galway Prison, 1921 (National Archives, Bishop Street, Dublin, Ireland).

Grant of Administration (Adeline English) 17 July 1944 (National Archives, Bishop Street, Dublin, Ireland).

Marriage Certificate, Patrick English and Honora Mulvihill, 18 February 1873 (General Register Office/An tSeirbhís um Chlárú Sibhialta, Roscommon, Ireland).

Medical Directory for 1905 (London: J. & A. Churchill, 1905).

Minutes of the Proceedings of the Committee of Management of Ballinasloe District Lunatic Asylum/Mental Hospital, 1904–1942 (Archives at St Brigid's Hospital, Ballinasloe, County Galway, Ireland).

Minutes of the Meeting of the Commissioner Administering the Affairs of the Ballinasloe Mental Hospital, 1940 (Archives at St Brigid's Hospital, Ballinasloe, County Galway, Ireland).

Minutes of Proceedings of the Commissioner Acting for the Dissolved Committee of Management of Ballinasloe Mental Hospital, 1940 (Archives at St Brigid's Hospital, Ballinasloe, County Galway, Ireland).

Official Report of Dáil Éireann (Houses of Oireachtas, Dublin, Ireland).

Official Report of Seanad Éireann (Houses of Oireachtas, Dublin, Ireland).

Schedule of Assets (Adeline English) 17 July 1944 (National Archives, Bishop Street, Dublin, Ireland).

Scoil Éanna Ltd Share Certificate, No. 31, 22 January 1912, PMSTE.2003.864 (Pearse Museum/OPW, St Enda's Park, Grange Road, Rathfarnham, County Dublin, Ireland).

Sworn Inquiry: Death of Patient (L2/102) (1927) HLTH/SL2/98 (National Archives, Bishop Street, Dublin, Ireland).

Sworn Inquiry: Death of Patient by Drowning (L2/102) (318/27) (22017/1939) HLTH/SL2/98 (National Archives, Bishop Street, Dublin, Ireland).

Sworn Inquiry: Request by Committee for Sworn Inquiry Re Management of Institution since 1934: Unfavourable Press Reports re Administration etc., Lack of Harmony between Officers of Institution (L2/102) (1940) HLTH/SL2/98 (National Archives, Bishop Street, Dublin, Ireland).

War Office 'Castle File No. 4168: Dr English, Ada' WO 35/206/75 (Kew, Richmond, Surrey: British National Archives).

Printed

Anonymous, 'Irish Division', *Journal of Mental Science*, 56, 235 (1910), p.776.

Anonymous, 'Ballinasloe Asylum', *Journal of Mental Science*, 62, 258 (1916), p.651.

Anonymous, 'Irish Division', *Journal of Mental Science*, 63, 263 (1917), p.620.

Anonymous, 'Medical news', *British Medical Journal*, 1, 1786 (1895), p.679.

Anonymous, 'Erratum', *British Medical Journal*, 1, 1787 (1895), p.738.

Anonymous, 'Book Notice: Tuberculosis in Children by Dorothy Stopford Price, MD', *Journal of the American Medical Association*, 140, 16 (1949), p.1308.

Boyd Barrett, E., 'Modern psycho-therapy and our asylums', *Studies*, 13, 49 (1924), pp.9–43.

Buckley, M., *The Jangle of the Keys* (Dublin: Duffy and Company, 1938).

Byrne, J.F., *Silent Years: An Autobiography with Memoirs of James Joyce and Our Ireland* (New York: Farrar, Strauss and Young, 1953).

Carbery, E., *The Four Winds of Eirinn: Poems by Ethna Carbery (Anna MacManus), Complete Edition* (Dublin: M. H. Gill and Son, Ltd 1906).

Dunne, J., 'Survey of modern physical methods of treatment for mental illness carried out in Grangegorman Mental Hospital', *Journal of the Medical Association of Eire*, 27, 157 (1950), pp.4–9.

Dunne, J., 'The contribution of the physical sciences to psychological medicine', *Journal of Mental Science*, 102, 427 (1956), pp.209–20.

Hallaran, W.S., *An Inquiry into the Causes producing the Extraordinary Addition to the Number of Insane together with Extended Observations on the Cure of Insanity with hints as to the Better Management of Public Asylums for Insane Persons* (Cork: Edwards and Savage, 1810).

Inspector of Lunatic Asylums in Ireland, *Report of the District, Local, and Private Lunatic Asylums in Ireland, 1846 (With Appendices)* (Dublin: Alexander Thom for Her Majesty's Stationery Office, 1847).

Inspectors of Lunatics, *The Forty-Second Report (With Appendices) of the Inspectors of Lunatics (Ireland)* (Dublin: Thom and Co. for Her Majesty's Stationery Office, 1893).

Kelly, B.D., 'Dr Ada English (1875–1944); doctor, patriot, politician', *British Journal of Psychiatry*, 204, 1 (2014), 5.

Meduna, L.J. Von, 'Versuche über die biologische Beeinflussung des Aflaubes der Schizophrenie', *Zeitschrift für die gesamte Neurologie und Psychiatrie*, 152, 1 (1935), pp.235–62.

Our Correspondent, 'Ballinasloe Lunatic Asylum', *Journal of Mental Science*, 62, 257 (1916), p.467.

Price, D.S., 'Analysis of BCG vaccinations', *Irish Journal of Medical Science*, 29, 2 (1954), pp.56–64.

Psychiatrist, 'Insanity in Ireland', *The Bell*, 7, 4 (1944), pp.303–10.

Stopford Price, D., and H.F. MacAuley, *Tuberculosis in Childhood* (Bristol: John Wright, 1942).

Stopford Price, D. and H.F. MacAuley, *Tuberculosis in Childhood (Second Edition)* (Bristol: John Wright, 1948)

Newspapers

Aberdeen Daily Journal
Ballinasloe Life
Connacht Tribune
Connacht Sentinel
Derby Daily Telegraph
East Galway Democrat
Evening Telegraph - Dundee
Gloucester Citizen
Hull Daily Mail
Irish Independent
Irish Medical News
Irish Medical Times
Irish Nation (Éire)
Irish Press
Irish Times
New York Times
Nottingham Evening Post
Poblacht na hÉireann: War News
Roscommon Champion
Roscommon Herald
Sunday Independent
Sunday Post – Glasgow
The Times
Western Daily Press – Bristol
Western News and Galway Leader
Western Times – Exeter

Periodicals

St Stephen's (college magazine of the Catholic University, Dublin)
Journal of Mental Science (journal of the Medico-Psychological Association of
Great Britain and Ireland)

Interviews

Finnerty, Mr Peter, Kiltormer, County Galway (interview in Ballinasloe,
Country Galway on 3 May 2013).
Hanniffy, Dr, Liam, Assistant Inspector of Mental Hospitals (retired) and son
of Mr John Hanniffy, assistant land steward, Mental Hospital, Ballinasloe,
County Galway (interview in Portlaoise, County Laois, 27 May 2013).
Illingworth, Councillor Ruth, historian (interview in Mullingar, County
Westmeath, 23 June 2013).
Murphy, Ms Joan Patricia, first cousin (once removed) of English (interview in
Ballinasloe, County Galway on 3 May 2013).

Secondary Sources

Barrington, R., *Health, Medicine and Politics in Ireland, 1900–1970* (Dublin:
Institute of Public Administration, 1987).
Bewley, T., *Madness to Mental Illness: A History of the Royal College of Psychiatrists*
(London: Royal College of Psychiatrists, 2008).
Brück, M., 'Torch-bearing women astronomers', in M. Mulvihill (ed.), *Lab
Coats and Lace: The Lives and Legacies of Inspiring Irish Women Scientists and
Pioneers* (Dublin: Women in Technology and Science, 2009), pp.73–85.
Carlson, E.T. and N. Dain, 'The psychotherapy that was moral treatment',
American Journal of Psychiatry, 117 (1960), pp.519–24.
Cherry, S. and R. Munting, '"Exercise is the thing": Sport and the asylum c1850–
1950', *International Journal of the History of Sport*, 22, 1 (2006), pp.42–58.
Clancy, M., 'On the "Western Outpost": Local government and women's
suffrage in county Galway', in G. Moran (ed.), *Galway: History and Society –
Interdisciplinary Essays on the History of an Irish County* (Dublin: Geography
Publications, 1996), pp.557–87.
Clancy, M., 'Shaping the Nation: Women in the Free State Parliament', in Y.
Galligan, E. Ward and R. Wilford (eds), *Contesting Politics: Women in Ireland,
North and South* (Boulder, Colorado: Westview Press, 1999), pp.201–18.
Clare, A. *Unlikely Rebels: The Gifford Girls and the Fight for Irish Freedom* (Dublin:
Mercier Press, 2011).

Clarke, F., 'English, Adeline ('Ada')', in J. McGuire and J. Quinn (eds), *Dictionary of Irish Biography: From the Earliest Times to the Year 2002 (Volume 3, D-F)* (Cambridge: Royal Irish Academy and Cambridge University Press, 2009), pp.626–7.

Clarke, K., (edited by H. Litton), *Revolutionary Woman: My Fight for Ireland's Freedom* (Dublin: The O'Brien Press, 1991).

Clear, C., *Nuns in Nineteenth-Century Ireland* (Dublin: Gill and Macmillan, 1987).

Collins, A., 'Eleonora Fleury captured', *British Journal of Psychiatry*, 203, 1 (2013), p.5.

Conlon, L., *Cumann na mBan and the Women of Ireland, 1913–1925* (Kilkenny: Kilkenny People Ltd, 1969).

Conolly Norman, J., *Richmond Asylum Joint Committee Minutes* (Dublin: Richmond Asylum, 1907), p.540.

Coogan, T.P., *Michael Collins: A Biography* (London: Arrow Books, 1991).

Coogan, T.P., *De Valera: Long Fellow, Long Shadow* (London: Hutchinson, 1993).

Cowell, J., *A Noontide Blazing: Brigid Lyons Thornton – Rebel, Soldier, Doctor* (Dublin: Currach Press, 2005).

Cox, C., *Negotiating Insanity in the Southeast of Ireland, 1820–1900* (Manchester and New York: Manchester University Press, 2012).

Davoren, M., E.G. Breen and B.D. Kelly, 'Dr Adeline English: revolutionising politics and psychiatry in Ireland', *Irish Psychiatrist*, 10, 4, (2009), pp. 260–2.

Davoren, M., E.G. Breen and B.D. Kelly, 'Dr Ada English: patriot and psychiatrist in early twentieth-century Ireland', *Irish Journal of Psychological Medicine*, 28, 2 (2011), pp.91–6.

Dudley Edwards, R., *Patrick Pearse: The Triumph of Failure* (Dublin: Irish Academic Press, 2006).

Dunne, O., '3rd Ada English Summer School', *Ballinasloe Life*, 3, 1 (April/May 2013), p.34.

Eichacker, J.M., *Irish Republican Women in America: Lecture Tours, 1916–1925* (Dublin: Irish Academic Press, 2007).

Ellman, R., *James Joyce (Second Edition)* (Oxford and New York: Oxford University Press, 1984).

Ferriter, D., *The Transformation of Ireland 1900–2000* (London: Profile Books, 2004).

Ferriter, D., *Judging Dev: A Reassessment of the Life and Legacy of Éamon de Valera* (Dublin: Royal Irish Academy, 2007).

Finnane, M., *Insanity and the Insane in Post-Famine Ireland* (London: Croom Helm, 1981).

Fitzgerald, E., 'There's women for you', *Irish Times*, 16 December 2000.

Fleetwood, J.F., *The History of Medicine in Ireland (Second Edition)* (Dublin: The Skellig Press, 1983).

Floate, S. and M. Harcourt Williams, 'Sketches from the history of psychiatry: "an innovation, a revolution" – the admission of women members to the Medico-Psychological Association', *Psychiatric Bulletin*, 15, 1 (1991), pp.28–30.

Fogarty, W., *Dr Eamonn O'Sullivan: A Man Before His Time* (Dublin: Wolfhound Press, 2007).

Foley, C., *The Last Irish Plague: The Great Flu Epidemic in Ireland, 1918–19* (Dublin: Irish Academic Press, 2011).

Fox, R.M., 'The Irish Citizen Army', in B. Ó Conchubhair (ed.), *Dublin's Fighting Story 1916–1921, Told By The Men Who Made It* (Dublin: Mercier Press, 2009), pp.52–9.

Fox, R.M. 'Citizen Army posts', in B. Ó Conchubhair (ed.), *Dublin's Fighting Story 1916–1921, Told By The Men Who Made It* (Dublin: Mercier Press, 2009), pp.107–17.

Fox, R.M., 'How the women helped', in B. Ó Conchubhair (ed.), *Dublin's Fighting Story 1916–1921, Told By The Men Who Made It* (Dublin: Mercier Press, 2009), pp.395–405.

Foy, M.T. and B. Barton, *The Easter Rising* (Dublin: Sutton Publishing, 2004).

Fuller Torrey, E. and J. Miller, *The Invisible Plague: The Rise of Mental Illness from 1750 to the Present* (New Brunswick, NJ and London: Rutgers University Press, 2001).

Greaves, C.D,. *Liam Mellows and the Irish Revolution* (Belfast: An Ghlór Gafa, 2004).

Griffith, A., *The Resurrection of Hungary: A Parallel for Ireland* (Dublin: Patrick Mahon, 1904).

Gueret, M., 'A lovely idea', *Sunday Independent*, 17 July 2011.

Harford, J., *The Opening of University Education to Women in Ireland* (Dublin: Irish Academic Press, 2007).

Healy, D., 'Irish psychiatry in the twentieth century', in G.E. Berrios and H. Freeman (eds), *150 Years of British Psychiatry. Volume II: The Aftermath* (London: Athlone Press, London, 1996), pp.268–91.

Healy D., 'Irish psychiatry. Part 2: Use of the Medico-Psychological Association by its Irish members-plus ca change!', in G.E. Berrios and H. Freeman (eds), *150 Years of British Psychiatry, 1841–1991* (London: Gaskell/Royal College of Psychiatrists, 1991), pp.314–20.

Henry, M., 'Medical women in parliament', *Irish Medical News*, 30 January 2001.

Hopkinson, M., *The Irish War of Independence* (Dublin: Gill and Macmillan Limited, 2004).

Illingworth, R., *Mullingar: History and Guide* (Dublin: Nonsuch, 2007).

Inspectors of Lunatics (Ireland), *The Forty-Second Report (With Appendices) of the Inspectors of Lunatics (Ireland) 1892* (Dublin: Alexander Thom and Company (Limited) for Her Majesty's Stationery Office, 1893).

Inspector of Mental Health Services, *Report of the Inspector of Mental Health Services 2011* (Dublin: Mental Health Commission, 2012).

Jones, G., 'The Campaign Against Tuberculosis in Ireland, 1899–1914', in E. Malcolm and G. Jones (eds), *Medicine, Disease and the State in Ireland, 1650–1940* (Cork: Cork University Press, 1999), pp.158–76.

Kearns, G., 'Mother Ireland and the revolutionary sisters', *Cultural Geographies*, 11, 4 (2004), pp.443–67.

Kelly, B., 'Female pioneers', *Irish Medical News*, 27 April 2009.

Kelly, B., 'The history of medicine', *Irish Medical News*, 8 August 2010.

Kelly, B., 'Irish women in medicine', *Irish Medical News*, 7 May 2013.

Kelly, B. and M. Davoren, 'Dr Ada English', in M. Mulvihill (ed.), *Lab Coats and Lace: The Lives and Legacies of Inspiring Irish Women Scientists and Pioneers* (Dublin: Women in Technology and Science, 2009), p.97.

Kelly, B.D., 'Mental illness in nineteenth-century Ireland: a qualitative study of workhouse records', *Irish Journal of Medical Science*, 173, 1 (2004), pp.53–5.

Kelly, B.D., 'Physical sciences and psychological medicine: the legacy of Prof John Dunne', *Irish Journal of Psychological Medicine*, 22, 2 (2005), pp.67–72.

Kelly, B.D., 'Structural violence and schizophrenia', *Social Science and Medicine*, 61, 3 (2005), pp.721–30.

Kelly, B.D., 'The power gap: freedom, power and mental illness', *Social Science and Medicine*, 63, 8 (2006), pp.2118–28.

Kelly, B.D., 'Ireland's Mental Health Act 2001', *Psychiatric Bulletin*, 31, 1 (2007), pp.21–4.

Kelly, B.D., 'One hundred years ago: the Richmond Asylum, Dublin in 1907', *Irish Journal of Psychological Medicine*, 24, 3 (2007), pp.108–14.

Kelly, B.D., 'Learning disability and forensic mental healthcare in nineteenth-century Ireland', *Irish Journal of Psychological Medicine*, 25, 3 (2008), pp.116–18.

Kelly, B.D., 'Mental health law in Ireland, 1821 to 1902: building the asylums', *Medico-Legal Journal*, 76, 1 (2008), pp.19–25.

Kelly, B.D., 'Mental health law in Ireland, 1821 to 1902: dealing with the "increase of insanity in Ireland"', *Medico-Legal Journal*, 7, 1 (2008), pp.26–33.

Kelly, B.D., 'The Mental Treatment Act 1945 in Ireland: an historical Inquiry', *History of Psychiatry*, 19, 1 (2008), pp.47–67.

Kelly, B.D., 'Dr William Saunders Hallaran and psychiatric practice in nineteenth-century Ireland', *Irish Journal of Medical Science*, 177, 1 (2008), pp.79–84.

Kelly, B.D., 'Criminal insanity in nineteenth-century Ireland, Europe and the United States: cases, contexts and controversies', *International Journal of Law and Psychiatry*, 32, 6 (2009), pp.362–8.

Kelly, B.D., 'Intellectual disability, mental illness and offending behaviour: forensic cases from early twentieth century Ireland', *Irish Journal of Medical Science*, 179, 3 (2010), pp.409–16.

Kelly, B.D., 'Tuberculosis in the nineteenth-century asylum: Clinical cases from the Central Criminal Lunatic Asylum, Dundrum, Dublin', in P.M. Prior (ed.), *Asylums, Mental Health Care and the Irish, 1800–2010* (Dublin: Irish Academic Press, 2011), pp.205–20.

Kelly, B.D., 'Mental illness and structural violence', *Irish Medical Journal*, 105, 1 (2012), p.30.

Kelly, D., *Between the Lines of History: People of Ballinasloe, Volume 1* (Ballinasloe: Declan Kelly, 2000).

Kelly, D. *Meadow of the Miracles: A History of the Diocese of Clonfert* (Strasbourg: Editions du Signe, 2006).

Kelly, D., *Ballinasloe: From Garbally Park to the Fairgreen* (Dublin: Nonsuch, 2007).

Kelly, L., *Irish Women in Medicine, c. 1880s–1920s: Origins, Education and Careers* (Manchester and New York: Manchester University Press, 2012).

Knirk, J., *Women of the Dáil: Gender, Republicanism and the Anglo-Irish Treaty* (Dublin: Irish Academic Press, 2006).

Lavelle, P., *James O'Mara: The Story of an Original Sinn Féiner* (Ireland: The History Publisher, 2011).

Lindsay, J.M., 'Presidential address delivered at the Fifty-Second Annual Meeting of the Medico-Psychological Association, held at the Palace Hotel, Buxton, 28 July, 1893', *Journal of Mental Science*, 39, 167 (1893), pp.473–91.

Lyons, F.S.L., *Ireland Since the Famine* (London: Fontana, 1985).

MacCurtain, M., *Ariadne's Thread: Writing Women into Irish History* (Galway: Arlen House, 2008).

Macken, M.M., 'Women in the University and the College: a struggle within a struggle', in M. Tierney (ed.), *Struggle with Fortune: A Miscellany for the Centenary of the Catholic University of Ireland, 1854–1954* (Dublin: Browne and Nolan, 1954), pp.142–65.

Mac Lellan, A., 'Dr Dorothy Price and the eradication of TB in Ireland', *Irish Medical News*, 19 May 2008.

Mac Lellan, A., 'Revolutionary doctors', in M. Mulvihill (ed.), *Lab Coats and Lace: The Lives and Legacies of Inspiring Irish Women Scientists and Pioneers* (Dublin: Women in Technology and Science, 2009), pp.86–101.

Mac Lellan, A., *Dorothy Stopford Price: Rebel Doctor* (Sallins, Co. Kildare: Irish Academic Press, 2014).

MacLoughlin, T., *Ballinasloe Inniú agus Inné: A Story of a Community Over the Past 300 Years* (Ballinasloe: Tadgh Mac Loughlin, 1993).

MacHale, D. and A. Mac Lellan, 'The fabulous Boole sisters', in M. Mulvihill (ed.), *Lab Coats and Lace: The Lives and Legacies of Inspiring Irish Women Scientists and Pioneers* (Dublin: Women in Technology and Science, 2009), pp.61–71.

Macleod, S.M. and H.N. McCullough, 'Social science education as a component of medical training', *Social Science and Medicine*, 39, 9 (November 1994), pp.1367–73.

Madden, J., *Fr John Fahy: Radical Republican and Agrarian Activist (1893–1969)* (Dublin: Columbia Press, 2012).

Matthews, A., *Dissidents: Irish Republican Women, 1923–1941* (Cork: Mercier Press, 2012).

Matthews, A., *Renegades: Irish Republican Women, 1900–1922* (Cork: Mercier Press, 2010).

McAuley, F., *Insanity, Psychiatry and Criminal Responsibility* (Dublin: Round Hall Press, 1993).

McCabe, A. and Mulholland, C. 'The red flag over the asylum: The Monaghan Asylum soviet of 1919', in P.M. Prior (ed.), *Asylums, Mental Health Care and the Irish, 1800–2010* (Dublin: Irish Academic Press, 2011), pp.23–43.

McCandless, P., 'Curative asylum, custodial hospital: The South Carolina Lunatic Asylum and State Hospital, 1828–1920', in R. Porter and D. Wright (eds), *The Confinement of the Insane: International Perspectives, 1800–1965* (Cambridge: Cambridge University Press, 2003), pp.173–92.

McCarthy, C., *Cumann na mBan and the Irish Revolution* (Dublin: The Collins Press, 2007).

McCoole, S., *No Ordinary Women: Irish Female Activists in the Revolutionary Years, 1900–1923* (Dublin: O'Brien Press, 2003).

McCrae, N., 'A violent thunderstorn: Cardiazol treatment in British mental hospitals', *History of Psychiatry*, 17, 1 (2006), pp.67–90.

McNamara, M. and P. Mooney, *Women in Parliament: 1918–2000* (Dublin: Wolfhound Press, 2000).

Meenan, F.O.C., *Cecilia Street: The Catholic University School of Medicine, 1855–1931* (Dublin: Gill and Macmillan, 1987).

Millon, T., *Masters of the Mind: Exploring the Story of Mental Illness from Ancient Times to the New Millennium* (Hoboken, NJ: John Wiley and Sons, 2004).

Mooney Eichacker, J., *Irish Republican Women in America: Lecture Tours, 1916–1925* (Dublin: Irish Academic Press, 2003).

Moore, R., 'Inaugural Ada English Symposium planned', *Ballinasloe Life*, 1 (2011), p.29.

Mulholland, M., *The Politics and Relationships of Kathleen Lynn* (Dublin: The Woodfield Press, 2002).

Mulvany, I., 'The Intermediate Act and the education of girls', *Irish Educational Review*, 1 (1907), pp.14–20.

Murray, J.P., *Galway: A Medico-Social History* (Galway: Kenny's Bookshop and Art Gallery, 1996).

O'Connell. C., 'First in their field', in M. Mulvihill (ed.), *Lab Coats and Lace: The Lives and Legacies of Inspiring Irish Women Scientists and Pioneers* (Dublin: Women in Technology and Science, 2009), pp.37–47.

O'Connor, A., 'Forget gender quotas, we need more Brigids in Dáil', *Irish Independent*, 12 May 2012.

O'Connor, U., 'Let's honour the father of Irish boxing', *Sunday Independent*, 26 August 2012.

O'Dubhghaill, S., 'Activities in Enniscorthy', *The Capuchin Annual*, 1966.

Ó hÓgartaigh, M., 'Dorothy Stopford Price and the elimination of childhood tuberculosis' in J. Augusteijn (ed.), *Ireland in the 1930s: New Perspectives* (Dublin: Four Courts Press, 1999), pp.67–82.

Ó hÓgartaigh, M., 'Women in university education in Ireland: the historical background' in A. Macdona (ed.), *From Newman to New Woman: UCD Women Remember* (Dublin: New Island Books, 2001), pp.iii–xi.

Ó hÓgartaigh, M., '"Is there any need of you?" Women in medicine in Ireland and Australia', *Australian Journal of Irish Studies*, 4 (2004), pp.162–71.

Ó hÓgartaigh, M., *Kathleen Lynn: Irishwoman, Patriot, Doctor* (Dublin: Irish Academic Press, 2006).

Ó hÓgartaigh, M., 'A quiet revolution: Irish women and second-level education, 1878–1930', *New Hibernia Review*, 13, 2 (2009), pp.36–51.

Ó hÓgartaigh, M., *Quiet Revolutionaries: Irish Women in Education, Medicine and Sport, 1861–1964* (Dublin: The History Press Ireland, 2011).

O'Neill, A.-M., *Irish Mental Health Law* (Dublin: First Law Ltd, 2005).

O'Sullivan, E.N.M., *Textbook of Occupational Therapy: With Chief Reference to Psychological Medicine* (Oxford: Philosophical Library, 1955).

Ó Broin, L., *Protestant Nationalists in Revolutionary Ireland: The Stopford Connection* (Dublin: Goldenbridge, 1985).

Plunkett Dillon, G. (edited by H. O Brolchain), *All in the Blood: A Memoir of the Plunkett Family, the 1916 Rising and the War of Independence* (Dublin: A. & A. Farmar, 2006).

Prior, P., 'Dangerous lunacy: The misuse of mental health law in nineteenth-century Ireland', *Journal of Forensic Psychiatry and Psychology*, 14, 3 (2003), pp.525–41.

Prior, P. (ed.), *Asylums, Mental Health Care and the Irish, 1800-2010* (Dublin: Irish Academic Press, 2012).

Reuber, M., 'The architecture of moral management: the Irish asylums (1801–1922)', *Psychological Medicine*, 26, 6 (1996), pp.1179–89.

Reynolds, J., *Grangegorman: Psychiatric Care in Dublin since 1815* (Dublin: Institute of Public Administration in association with Eastern Health Board, 1992).

Rivington, W., *The Medical Profession* (Dublin: Fannin and Company, 1879).

Robins, J., *Fools and Mad: A History of the Insane in Ireland* (Dublin: Institute of Public Administration, 1986).

Sheridan, A.J., 'The impact of political transition on psychiatric nursing – a case study of twentieth-century Ireland', *Nursing Inquiry*, 13, 4 (2006), pp. 289–299.

Shorter, E., *A History of Psychiatry: From the Era of the Asylum to the Age of Prozac* (New York: John Wiley & Sons, 1997).

Shorter, E. and D. Healy, *Shock Therapy: A History of Electroconvulsive Treatment in Mental Illness* (New Brunswick, NJ and London: Rutgers University Press, 2007).

Smith, L.D., 'The county asylum in the mixed economy of care, 1808–1845', in J. Melling and B. Forsythe (eds), *Insanity Institutions and Society, 1800–1914: A Social History of Madness in Comparative Perspective* (London and New York: Routledge, 1999), pp.33–47.

Smith, L., *Lunatic Hospitals in Georgian England, 1750–1830 (Routledge Studies in the Social History of Medicine)* (London: Routledge, 2007).

Walsh, D., 'The ups and downs of schizophrenia in Ireland', *Irish Journal of Psychiatry*, 13, 2 (1992), pp.12–16.

Walsh, O., 'Gender and insanity in nineteenth-century Ireland', *Clio Medica / The Wellcome Series in the History of Medicine*, 73, 1 (2004), pp. 69–93.

Walsh, O., '"Tales from the big house": The Connacht District Lunatic Asylum in the late nineteenth century', *History Ireland*, 13, 6 (2005), pp.21–5.

Walsh, O., 'A perfectly ordered establishment: Connaught District Lunatic Asylum (Ballinasloe)', in P.M. Prior (ed.), *Asylums, Mental Health Care and the Irish, 1800–2010* (Dublin: Irish Academic Press, 2011), pp.246–70.

Walsh, O., 'Cure or Custody: Therapeutic Philosophy at the Connaught District Lunatic Asylum', in M.H. Preston and M. Ó hÓgartaigh (eds), *Gender and Medicine in Ireland, 1700–1950* (Syracuse, NY: Syracuse University Press, 2012), pp.69–85.

Walsh, D. and A. Daly, *Mental Illness in Ireland, 1750–2002: Reflections on the Rise and Fall of Institutional Care* (Dublin: Health Research Board, 2004).

Ward, M., *Unmanageable Revolutionaries: Women in Irish Nationalism* (London: Pluto Press, 1995).

Ward, M., 'Times of transition: Republican women, feminism and political representation', in L. Ryan and M. Ward (eds), *Irish Women and Nationalism: Soldiers, New Women and Wicked Hags* (Dublin: Irish Academic Press, 2004), pp.184–201.

Williamson, A., 'The beginnings of state care for the mentally ill in Ireland', *Economic and Social Review (Ireland)*, 10, 1 (1970), pp.280–91.

Wyse Jackson, P.N., 'Erratics, intrusions and graptolites', in M. Mulvihill (ed.), *Lab Coats and Lace: The Lives and Legacies of Inspiring Irish Women Scientists and Pioneers* (Dublin: Women in Technology and Science, 2009), pp.49–59.

INDEX